Anesthesia Outside the Operating Room

Editors

MARK S. WEISS
WENDY L. GROSS

ANESTHESIOLOGY CLINICS

www.anesthesiology.theclinics.com

Consulting Editor
LEE A. FLEISHER

December 2017 • Volume 35 • Number 4

ELSEVIER

1600 John F. Kennedy Boulevard • Suite 1800 • Philadelphia, Pennsylvania, 19103-2899

http://www.theclinics.com

ANESTHESIOLOGY CLINICS Volume 35, Number 4
December 2017 ISSN 1932-2275, ISBN-13: 978-0-323-54540-2

Editor: Colleen Dietzler
Developmental Editor: Kristen Helm

Anesthesiology Clinics (ISSN 1932-2275) is published quarterly by Elsevier Inc., 360 Park Avenue South, New York, NY 10010-1710. Months of issue are March, June, September, and December. Periodicals postage paid at New York, NY and at additional mailing offices. Subscription prices are $100.00 per year (US student/resident), $333.00 per year (US individuals), $404.00 per year (Canadian individuals), $620.00 per year (US institutions), $783.00 per year (Canadian institutions), $225.00 per year (Canadian and foreign student/resident), $460.00 per year (foreign individuals), and $783.00 per year (foreign institutions). To receive student and resident rate, orders must be accompanied by name of affiliated institution, date of term, and the *signature* of program/residency coordinator on institutions letterhead. Orders will be billed at individual rate until proof of status is received. Foreign air speed delivery is included in all *Clinics'* subscription prices. All prices are subject to change without notice. POSTMASTER: Send address changes to *Anesthesiology Clinics,* Elsevier Health Sciences Division, Subscription Customer Service, 3251 Riverport Lane, Maryland Heights, MO 63043. Customer Service (orders, claims, online, change of address): Elsevier Health Sciences Division, Subscription Customer Service, 3251 Riverport Lane, Maryland Heights, MO 63043. **Tel:1-800-654-2452 (U.S. and Canada); 314-447-8871 (outside U.S. and Canada). Fax: 314-447-8029. E-mail: journalscustomerservice-usa@elsevier. com (for print support); journalsonlinesupport-usa@elsevier.com (for online support).**

Reprints. For copies of 100 or more of articles in this publication, please contact the Commercial Reprints Department, Elsevier Inc., 360 Park Avenue South, New York, NY 10010-1710. Tel.: 212-633-3874; Fax: 212-633-3820; E-mail: reprints@elsevier.com.

Anesthesiology Clinics, is also published in Spanish by McGraw-Hill Inter-americana Editores S. A., P.O. Box 5-237, 06500 Mexico D. F., Mexico.

Anesthesiology Clinics, is covered in *MEDLINE/PubMed (Index Medicus), Current Contents/Clinical Medicine, Excerpta Medica, ISI/BIOMED,* and *Chemical Abstracts.*

Contributors

CONSULTING EDITOR

LEE A. FLEISHER, MD, FACC, FAHA
Robert D. Dripps Professor and Chair of Anesthesiology and Critical Care, Professor of Medicine, Perelman School of Medicine Health System, University of Pennsylvania, Philadelphia, Pennsylvania

EDITORS

MARK S. WEISS, MD
Assistant Professor of Anesthesiology and Critical Care, Director, Inpatient Endoscopy Anesthesia, Hospital of the University of Pennsylvania, Philadelphia, Pennsylvania

WENDY L. GROSS, MD, MHCM
Vice Chair, Planning and Analytics, Director, Non-OR Services, Faculty, Division of Cardiac Anesthesia, Department of Anesthesiology, Perioperative and Pain Medicine, Brigham and Women's Hospital, Boston, Massachusetts

AUTHORS

ANNIE AMIN, MD
Department of Anesthesiology, The University of Chicago, Chicago, Illinois

SAIF ANWARUDDIN, MD, FACC, FSCAI
Assistant Professor of Medicine, Perelman School of Medicine University of Pennsylvania, Co-Director, Transcatheter Valve Program, Hospital of the University of Pennsylvania, Philadelphia, Pennsylvania

PHILIP D. BAILEY Jr, DO, MBA
Assistant Professor, Department of Anesthesiology and Critical Care Medicine, Perelman School of Medicine University of Pennsylvania, The Children's Hospital of Philadelphia, Philadelphia, Pennsylvania

SHARATH K. BHAGAVATULA, MD
Department of Radiology, Brigham and Women's Hospital, Harvard Medical School, Boston, Massachusetts

STEVEN BOGGS, MD, FASA, MBA
Professor and Vice Chair, Clinical and Research Affairs, Department of Anesthesiology, University of Tennessee College of Medicine, UTHSC/Regional One Health, Memphis, Tennessee

JASON T. BOUHENGUEL, MD, MS
Anesthesiology Resident, Department of Anesthesiology, Perioperative and Pain Medicine, Brigham and Women's Hospital, Harvard Medical School, Boston, Massachusetts

VINAY CHANDRASEKHARA, MD,
Assistant Professor of Medicine, Gastroenterology Division, Perelman School of Medicine University of Pennsylvania, Philadelphia, Pennsylvania

LEBRON COOPER, MD, FASA
Professor and Chair, Department of Anesthesiology, University of Tennessee College of Medicine, UTHSC/Regional One Health, Memphis, Tennessee

THOMAS CUTTER, MD, MAEd
Department of Anesthesiology, The University of Chicago, Chicago, Illinois

DAVID M. DIBARDINO, MD
Assistant Professor of Clinical Medicine, Section of Interventional Pulmonology, Division of Pulmonary, Allergy and Critical Care, University of Pennsylvania, Philadelphia, Pennsylvania

KAREN B. DOMINO, MD, MPH
Professor and Vice Chair for Clinical Research, Department of Anesthesiology and Pain Medicine, University of Washington, Seattle, Washington

PAUL N. FIORILLI, MD
Fellow, Interventional Cardiology, Cardiovascular Division, Department of Anesthesiology and Critical Care, Hospital of the University of Pennsylvania, Philadelphia, Pennsylvania

DAVID S. FRANKEL, MD
Electrophysiology Section, Cardiovascular Division, Perelman School of Medicine University of Pennsylvania, Philadelphia, Pennsylvania

GREGORY G. GINSBERG, MD
Director of Endoscopic Services, Gastroenterology Division, Professor of Medicine, Perelman School of Medicine University of Pennsylvania, Penn Medicine, Abramson Cancer Center, Ruth & Raymond Perelman Center for Advanced Medicine, Philadelphia, Pennsylvania

BARBARA GOLD, MD, MS
Professor, Anesthesiology, Anesthesiology Administration, Executive Vice President Medical Affairs, University of Minnesota Health, Minneapolis, Minnesota

WENDY L. GROSS, MD, MHCM
Vice Chair, Planning and Analytics, Director, Non-OR Services, Faculty, Division of Cardiac Anesthesia, Department of Anesthesiology, Perioperative and Pain Medicine, Brigham and Women's Hospital, Boston, Massachusetts

ANDREW R. HAAS, MD, PhD
Associate Professor of Medicine, Section of Interventional Pulmonology, Division of Pulmonary, Allergy and Critical Care, University of Pennsylvania, Philadelphia, Pennsylvania

MICHAEL HALL, MD
Assistant Professor of Anesthesiology, Department of Anesthesiology and Critical Care, Hospital of the University of Pennsylvania, Philadelphia, Pennsylvania

HANSOL KIM, MD
Resident, Department of Radiology, Division of Angiography and Interventional Radiology, Brigham and Women's Hospital, Harvard Medical School, Boston, Massachusetts

MICHAEL L. KOCHMAN, MD, AGAF, FASGE
Wilmott Family Professor of Medicine, Director, Center for Endoscopic Innovation, Research, and Training, Gastroenterology Division, Perelman School of Medicine University of Pennsylvania, Philadelphia, Pennsylvania

JASON LANE, MD, MPH
Associate Professor of Clinical Anesthesiology, Associate Professor of Clinical Radiology and Radiological Sciences, Department of Anesthesiology, Vanderbilt University Medical Center, Nashville, Tennessee

MEGHAN B. LANE-FALL, MD, MSHP
Assistant Professor, Department of Anesthesiology and Critical Care, Perelman School of Medicine University of Pennsylvania, Philadelphia, Pennsylvania

KELLY LEBAK, MD
Senior Clinical Instructor, Case Western Reserve University School of Medicine, The MetroHealth System, Brecksville Ambulatory Surgery Center Medical Director, Cleveland, Ohio

JEFF E. MANDEL, MD, MS
Department of Anesthesiology and Critical Care, Perelman School of Medicine University of Pennsylvania, Philadelphia, Pennsylvania

SHIVAN J. MEHTA, MD, MBA
Assistant Professor, Division of Gastroenterology, Perelman School of Medicine University of Pennsylvania, Philadelphia, Pennsylvania

RICHARD C. MONTH, MD
Assistant Professor, Department of Anesthesiology and Critical Care, University of Pennsylvania, Philadelphia, Pennsylvania

OLIVIA NELSON, MD
Pediatric Anesthesiology Fellow, Department of Anesthesiology and Critical Care Medicine, The Children's Hospital of Philadelphia, Philadelphia, Pennsylvania

DAVID A. PREISS, MD, PhD
Assistant Professor, Department of Anesthesiology, Perioperative and Pain Medicine, Brigham and Women's Hospital, Harvard Medical School, Boston, Massachusetts

ROLF SCHLICHTER, MD
Associate Professor, Department of Anesthesiology and Critical Care, University of Pennsylvania, Hospital of the University of Pennsylvania, Philadelphia, Pennsylvania

JOHN P. SCOTT, MD
Director of Pediatric Liver Transplant Anesthesia, Associate Professor, Anesthesiology, Division of Pediatric Anesthesiology, Associate Professor, Pediatrics, Division of Pediatric Critical Care, Associate Medical Director, Pediatric Intensive Care Unit, Children's Hospital of Wisconsin, Medical College of Wisconsin, Milwaukee, Wisconsin

RONAK SHAH, MD
Assistant Professor, Adult Cardiothoracic Anesthesiology, Department of
Anesthesiology and Critical Care, Hospital of the University of Pennsylvania, Philadelphia,
Pennsylvania

CHRISTOPHER D. SHARP, MD, MS
Assistant Professor, Associate Medical Director of Outpatient Surgery, Center Director of
Medical Student Clerkship, The University of Tennessee Health Science Center,
Memphis, Tennessee

PAUL SHYN, MD
Department of Radiology, Brigham and Women's Hospital, Harvard Medical School,
Boston, Massachusetts

SHAZIA MEHMOOD SIDDIQUE, MD
Fellow, Division of Gastroenterology, Perelman School of Medicine University of
Pennsylvania, Philadelphia, Pennsylvania

MICHAEL S. STECKER, MD
Assistant Professor, Department of Radiology, Division of Angiography and Interventional
Radiology, Brigham and Women's Hospital, Harvard Medical School, Boston,
Massachusetts

WILLIAM G. STEVENSON, MD
Electrophysiology Section, Cardiovascular Division, Brigham and Women's Hospital,
Harvard Medical School, Boston, Massachusetts

RICHARD TAUS, MD
SMG Radiology, Morton Hospital, Taunton, Massachusetts

EZEKIEL TAYLER, DO
Intensivist, Anesthesiologist, Cardiothoracic ICU, Lankenau Medical Center,
Wynnewood, Pennsylvania

JOHN MICHAEL TRUMMEL, MD, MPH
Assistant Professor, Anesthesiology, Dartmouth-Hitchcock Medical Center, Lebanon,
New Hampshire

RICHARD D. URMAN, MD, MBA, FASA
Associate Professor, Department of Anesthesiology, Perioperative and Pain Medicine,
Brigham and Women's Hospital, Center for Perioperative Research, Brigham and
Women's Hospital, Harvard Medical School, Boston, Massachusetts

STYLIANOS VOULGARELIS, MD
Assistant Professor of Anesthesiology, Divisions of Pediatric and Adult Cardiac
Anesthesiology, Medical College of Wisconsin, Milwaukee, Wisconsin

MARK S. WEISS, MD
Assistant Professor of Anesthesiology and Critical Care, Director, Inpatient Endoscopy
Anesthesia, Hospital of the University of Pennsylvania, Philadelphia, Pennsylvania

ZACHARY G. WOODWARD, MD
Resident in Anesthesia, Department of Anesthesiology, Perioperative and Pain Medicine, Brigham and Women's Hospital, Harvard Medical School, Boston, Massachusetts

ELIZABETH ZHOU, MD
Assistant Professor, Adult Cardiothoracic Anesthesiology, Department of Anesthesiology and Critical Care, Hospital of the University of Pennsylvania, Philadelphia, Pennsylvania

Contents

Evolving financial and medical constraints fueled by the increasing repertoire of nonoperating room cases and widening scope of patient comorbidities are discussed. The need to integrate finances and care approaches is detailed, and strategic suggestions for broader collaborative practice are suggested.

Active maintenance of highly functional teams is critical to ensuring safe, efficient patient care in the non–operating room anesthesia (NORA) suite. In addition to developing collaborative relationships and patient care protocols, individual and team training is needed. For anesthesiologists, this training must begin during residency. The training should be supplemented with continuing education in this field for providers who find themselves working in the NORA space. As NORA continues to grow, robust NORA-specific quality assurance and improvement programs will empower anesthesiologists with the tools they need to best care for these patients.

Malpractice claims for non–operating room anesthesia care (NORA) had a higher proportion of claims for death than claims in operating rooms (ORs). NORA claims most frequently involved monitored anesthesia care. Inadequate oxygenation/ventilation was responsible for one-third of NORA claims, often judged probably preventable by better monitoring. Fewer malpractice claims for NORA occurred than for OR anesthesia as assessed by the relative numbers of NORA versus OR procedures. The proportion of claims in cardiology and radiology NORA locations was increased compared with estimates of cases in these locations. Although NORA is safe, adherence to safe clinical practice is important.

Non–operating room anesthesia (NORA) encounters comprise a significant fraction of contemporary anesthesia practice. With the implementation of an anesthesia information management system (AIMS), anesthesia practitioners can better streamline preoperative assessment, intraoperative automated documentation, real-time decision support, and remote surveillance. Despite the large personal and financial commitments involved in adoption and implementation of AIMS and other electronic health records in these settings, the benefits to safety, efficacy, and efficiency are far too great to be ignored. Continued future innovation of AIMS technology only promises to further improve on our NORA experience and improve care quality and safety.

Procedures requiring nonoperating room anesthesia (NORA) continue to increase in quantity and complexity. The roles of anesthesiologists as members of care teams in nonoperating room locations continue to evolve. The safe provision of NORA requires strict adherence to standardized monitoring guidelines, including pulse oximetry, capnography, electrocardiogram, and noninvasive blood pressure amplifier. Body temperature also should be measured in appropriate scenarios. High-risk anesthetics require advanced preparation and monitoring.

In the setting of technological advancements in imaging and intervention with concomitant rise in the use of non–operating room anesthesia (NORA) care, it has become even more critical for anesthesiologists to be aware of the needs and limitations of interventional procedures performed outside of the operating room. This article addresses the use of NORA services from the interventional radiologist's point of view and provides specific examples of preprocedural, intraprocedural, and postprocedural care patients may need for optimal outcome.

The advent of radiology image–guided tumor ablation procedures has opened a new era in minimally invasive procedures. Using computed tomography, MRI, ultrasound, and other modalities, radiologists and surgeons can now ablate a tumor through percutaneous entry sites. What traditionally was done in an operating room via large open incisions, with multiple days in the hospital recovering, is now becoming an outpatient procedure via these new techniques. Anesthesiologists play a critical role in optimizing outcome in these patients. Knowledge by anesthesiologists of procedural goals, technology used, and inherent safety concerns of anesthetizing patients in the radiology suite are all critical to patients and proceduralists.

Sharath K. Bhagavatula, Jason Lane, and Paul Shyn

Image-guided percutaneous, minimally invasive ablation techniques offer a wide variety of new modalities to treat tumors in some of the most medically complicated patients coming to our hospitals. The use of computed tomography, PET, ultrasound imaging, and MRI to guide radio-frequency ablation, microwave ablation, and cryoablation techniques now makes it possible to treat patients on a short stay or outpatient basis with very good immediate outcomes. This rapid expansion of new tumor ablation techniques often presents challenges for the non–operating room anesthesia team. Collaboration and communication between the radiologist and anesthesiologist are key to safety and excellent patient outcomes.

Paul N. Fiorilli, Saif Anwaruddin, Elizabeth Zhou, and Ronak Shah

The cardiac catheterization laboratory is advancing medicine by performing procedures on patients who would usually require sternotomy and cardiopulmonary bypass. These procedures are done percutaneously, allowing them to be performed on patients considered inoperable. Patients have compromised cardiovascular function or advanced age. An anesthesiologist is essential for these procedures in case of hemodynamic compromise. Interventionalists are becoming more familiar with transcatheter aortic valve replacement and the device has become smaller, both contributing to fewer complications. Left atrial occlusion and the endovascular edge-to-edge mitral valve repair devices were approved. Although these devices require general anesthesia, an invasive surgery and cardiopulmonary bypass machine are not necessary for deployment.

Jeff E. Mandel, William G. Stevenson, and David S. Frankel

 Video content accompanies this article at http://www.anesthesiology. theclinics.com.

The electrophysiology suite is a foreign location to many anesthesiologists. The initial experience was with shorter procedures under conscious sedation, and the value of greater tailoring of the sedation/anesthesia by anesthesiologists was not perceived until practice patterns had already been established. Although better control of ventilation with general anesthesia may be expected, suppression of arrhythmias, blunting of the hemodynamic adaptation to induced arrhythmias, and interference by muscle relaxants with identification of the phrenic nerve may be seen. We review a range of electrophysiology procedures and discuss anesthetic approaches that balance patient safety and favorable outcomes.

Patients with atrial fibrillation and flutter routinely require transesophageal echocardiography with cardioversion. It is not uncommon to encounter patients with reduced ejection fractions, coronary artery disease, prior cardiac surgery, or obstructive sleep apnea. The anesthesiologist must carefully evaluate the patient and any available laboratory and study findings to assess for potential complications after anesthesia. Appropriate anesthetics must be chosen based on the preoperative evaluation. Additionally, because most of these cases are done without a secured airway, emergency medications and airway equipment must be readily available.

This article aims to detail the breadth and depth of advanced upper gastrointestinal endoscopic procedures. It focuses on sedation and airway management concerns pertaining to this emerged and emerging class of minimally invasive interventions. The article also covers endoscopic hemostasis, endoscopic resection, stenting, and Barrett eradication therapy plus endoscopic ultrasound. It additionally addresses the nuances of endoscopic retrograde cholangiopancreatography and new natural orifice transluminal endoscopic surgery procedures, including endoscopic cystogastrostomy and the per-oral endoscopic myotomy procedure.

Demand for anesthesiologist-assisted sedation is expanding for gastrointestinal lower endoscopic procedures and may add to the cost of these procedures. Most lower endoscopy procedures can be accomplished with either no, moderate, or deep sedation; general anesthesia and active airway management are rarely needed. Propofol-based sedation has advantages in terms of satisfaction and recovery over other modalities, but moderate sedation using benzodiazepines and opiates work well for low-risk patients and procedures. No sedation for routine colonoscopy works well for selected patients and eliminates sedation-related risks. There is no difference in outcome measures based on sedation received.

Bronchoscopy presents a unique challenge and need for collaboration between anesthesia providers and bronchoscopists. The approach to topical anesthesia, analgesia, and sedation must be customized based on complexity, duration, and setting. The bronchoscopy team must work together in each phase of the procedure to ensure patient safety and allow completion of a quality bronchoscopy. Airway access may change depending on the type of procedure planned and must be discussed before each case. Intraprocedural difficulties with ventilation, airway pressure, and sedation may arise that must be addressed together. This review highlights an approach to these common challenges.

Olivia Nelson and Philip D. Bailey Jr

Anesthesiologists are increasingly called on to care for pediatric patients undergoing diagnostic imaging and invasive procedures in interventional radiology. These procedures are typically classified as either nonvascular or vascular, and can range from short diagnostic imaging studies or biopsies to significantly longer and more invasive intravascular procedures. Anesthesia providers must consider each child's ability to cooperate reliably during the procedure, the child's age, and any cognitive impairment to define the best anesthetic plan. Several unique pediatric patient populations with specific procedural implications and anesthetic considerations who will benefit from additional periprocedural planning are discussed.

Shazia Mehmood Siddique and Shivan J. Mehta

To control costs and improve quality, changes in health care delivery and financing have emerged, resulting in shifting of financial risk to providers for the quality and cost of care, including emergence of accountable care organizations and bundled payment models. This article discusses health care financing and delivery models in the context of procedures and surgeries that happen outside of the operating room. It describes the history of health insurance, trends in ambulatory surgery centers, and new payment models that have emerged from the Affordable Care Act and the Medicare Access and Children's Health Insurance Program Reauthorization Act.

Wendy L. Gross, Lebron Cooper, Steven Boggs, and Barbara Gold

The anesthesia market continues to undergo disruption. Financial margins are shrinking, and buyers are demanding that anesthesia services be provided in an efficient, low-cost manner. To help anesthesiologists analyze their market, Drucker and Porter's framework of buyers, suppliers, quality, barriers to entry, substitution, and strategic priorities allows for a structured analysis. Once this analysis is completed, anesthesiologists must articulate their value to other medical professionals and to hospitals. Anesthesiologists can survive and thrive in a value-based health care environment if they are capable of providing services differently and are able to deliver cost-effective care.

ANESTHESIOLOGY CLINICS

RELATED INTEREST

Gastrointestinal Endoscopy Clinics of North America, July 2016 (Vol. 26, No. 3)
Sedation and Monitoring in Gastrointestinal Endoscopy
John J. Vargo, *Editor*
Available at: http://www.giendo.theclinics.com/

THE CLINICS ARE AVAILABLE ONLINE!
Access your subscription at:
www.theclinics.com

Foreword

Anesthesia Outside of the Operating Room: The Wild West or the New Frontier?

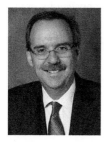

Lee A. Fleisher, MD, FACC, FAHA
Consulting Editor

An ever-increasing percentage of anesthetics is being performed outside of the operating room (OR) setting. These cases initially represented a small part of our care, but with the development of minimally invasive medical procedures, we are spending more time outside the OR. While outpatient endoscopy represents a procedure in healthy individuals that can also be effectively performed with sedation, some of the newer procedures are performed in those with multiple comorbidities and require significant anesthetic skill. Understanding the logistics of providing such care outside of our usual comfort zone of the OR is the topic of the current issue of the *Anesthesiology Clinics*.

This issue was proposed by two leaders in thought in this arena, Mark S. Weiss, MD and Wendy L. Gross, MD. Dr Weiss is Assistant Professor of Anesthesiology and Critical Care at the University of Pennsylvania. He directs the inpatient endoscopy anesthesia service at Penn and is developing an online educational platform, NORAlink. Dr Gross is Assistant Professor of Anesthesiology, Perioperative and Pain Medicine at Harvard Medical School and Director of the Cardiac Anesthesia Liaison Service at Brigham and Women's Hospital. Dr Gross is the President of SONORIA, the Society of Non-OR Intervention and Anesthesia. Together, they have brought together a

Anesthesiology Clin 35 (2017) xv–xvi
https://doi.org/10.1016/j.anclin.2017.09.002
1932-2275/17/© 2017 Published by Elsevier Inc.

phenomenal group of authors from both anesthesia and the relevant medical specialties to educate us on best current practices.

Lee A. Fleisher, MD, FACC, FAHA
Perelman School of Medicine Health System
University of Pennsylvania
3400 Spruce Street, Dulles 680
Philadelphia, PA 19104, USA

E-mail address:
Lee.Fleisher@uphs.upenn.edu

Preface

Anesthesia Outside the Operating Room

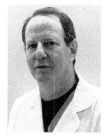 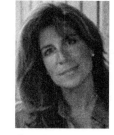

Mark S. Weiss, MD   Wendy L. Gross, MD, MHCM
Editors

Shortly after I arrived at the University of Pennsylvania in 2011, I attended an early morning meeting of the Non-Operating Room Anesthesia (NORA) team. I had been in private practice for years, and only a few months earlier left that practice for Penn. It was as a private practice anesthesiologist that we first noticed these "Out-of-OR" cases. At first, there were only a few cases. However, over time, we were being asked to provide more services to outside areas that evoked discomfort on several levels. Among the issues that arose were: What is best for the NORA patient? How should we do these cases? What does the proceduralist need? How do we staff these services? Who pays for our time, expenses, monitors, and auxiliary staff? And when I came to Penn, I noticed rather quickly that these very same questions were being asked.

During that meeting of our Penn NORA team, we identified the upcoming surge of growth in NORA case volume. At that time, at Hospital of the University of Pennsylvania, about 6% of all our anesthesia cases occurred outside the OR. We predicted that in just a few years, more than 25% of our cases would involve NORA. (Today, we are actually doing over a third of cases in this manner.) I looked around the room and all I saw was the "Old Guard" of anesthesiologists. Being new to the department, I raised my hand and asked, "How are we training our residents for the future?" My colleagues' response was the following: "You know, we all learned how to do this on the fly…"

That is just not good enough.

Back in 2011, there were no defined "best practices" published. There was precious little direction for NORA cases nationally. The American Society of Anesthesiologists had published some recommendations, but no clear guidelines addressing what was required to care safely for patients in the NORA setting. We needed standards, guidelines, and teaching programs. In addition, economic issues needed to be

Anesthesiology Clin 35 (2017) xvii–xix
https://doi.org/10.1016/j.anclin.2017.09.001
1932-2275/17/© 2017 Published by Elsevier Inc.

addressed. Finally, ground rules for collaboration needed to be established to deal with the anticipated continued rise in NORA case volume.

To prepare for the future, it is helpful to examine the reasons that led to how you arrived at the present. There are several large "tectonic plates" acting as driving forces behind the groundswell of growth in NORA: an aging population with multiple medical comorbidities; the service expectations of both health care consumers and providers; cost and value for insurance companies, health care institutions, and government; and advances in various procedural techniques have resulted in continued improvements and expansion in NORA. Today, anesthesia teams are coordinating and collaborating with proceduralists from various specialties to develop standards and practices to ensure patient safety as well as the success of procedures. Anesthesiologists are involved in all aspects of the care of NORA patients throughout the hospital in multiple clinical settings.

This issue of the *Anesthesiology Clinics* is only a snapshot of NORA in time. Although our field has made progress, I believe that the evolution of NORA in the coming years will revolutionize the way medicine is delivered in this country, and that we will look back at this issue in several years and be pleasantly surprised at how this field has evolved. It seems as if almost every day a new procedure is demonstrated or a new technique is developed. The opportunity for improved and efficient health care is changing rapidly thanks to the innovative, collaborative, imaginative minds and efforts of those involved.

The issues and topics covered in this issue are as varied as NORA itself. When we discussed how to organize this effort, Wendy Gross and I agreed that when possible the articles in this project, just as in the NORA suite, would be a collaborative effort by an anesthesiologist and a proceduralist expert in their respective field. The results of these collaborations were a fascinating series of articles focusing on different and important aspects of NORA. This issue includes thoughtful discussions on the changing landscape of NORA care, organization, and information systems. In addition, there are interesting reviews of safety in the NORA suite using closed claims data and monitoring. Clinically, a variety of settings and procedures are examined. One procedure in particular, tumor ablation in the radiology suite, is closely examined from the view of both the anesthesia team and the radiologist, allowing us to look at our field from our colleagues' perspective. Finally, in recognition of the economic implications of the growth of NORA, we have included a section regarding market evaluation on finances, bundled payments, and Accountable Care Organizations, as well as how to plan and strategize priorities for the future.

Wendy and I would like to thank the many contributors among multiple institutions from many specialties who have contributed to the success of this project. We are thankful to Dr Lee Fleisher, Professor and Chairman of Anesthesiology at the University of Pennsylvania, for giving us the opportunity to edit this issue of the *Anesthesiology Clinics*, and to the professionals at Elsevier for their encouragement and advice with this endeavor. We are especially grateful to our families for their patience and understanding of the commitment of time that this project took to complete.

Mark S. Weiss, MD
Department of Anesthesiology and Critical Care
Hospital of the University of Pennsylvania
3400 Spruce Street
6th Floor Dulles Building
Philadelphia, PA 19104, USA

Wendy L. Gross, MD, MHCM
Division of Cardiac Anesthesia
Department of Anesthesiology, Perioperative and Pain Medicine
Brigham and Women's Hospital
75 Francis Street
Boston, MA 02115, USA

E-mail addresses:
weissm@uphs.upenn.edu; mweiss@sonoria.org (M.S. Weiss)
wgross@partners.org (W.L. Gross)

Demands of Integrated Care Delivery in Interventional Medicine and Anesthesiology

Interdisciplinary Teamwork and Strategy

Wendy L. Gross, MD, MHCM[a,*], Lebron Cooper, MD[b],
Steven Boggs, MD, MBA[b]

KEYWORDS

- Strategy • Nonoperating room anesthesia • Clinical operations anesthesia
- Integrated care delivery • Interventional medicine • Anesthesiology
- Interdisciplinary teamwork

KEY POINTS

- Evolving financial constraints for nonoperating room or services.
- New noninvasive approaches to treatment and implications for operations.
- Financial silos and implications for care integration.
- Increasing scope of patient comorbidities for nonoperating room patients.
- Collaborative practice for nonsurgeons and anesthesiologists.

There is no longer any doubt that the growing array of noninvasive procedures performed outside of the operating room offers substantial benefit and increased value over traditional surgical alternatives. Interventional medical procedures performed by cardiologists, gastroenterologists, pulmonologists, and radiologists now offer effective alternatives to traditional surgery.[1]

In fact, nonoperating room procedural volume exceeds operating room surgical case volume in many hospitals.[2] As volume grows, the scope of cases expands as well. Older and more complex patients increasingly undergo technically sophisticated treatments performed in procedural suites with the support of anesthesiologists.[3]

Disclosure Statement: No disclosures.
[a] Division of Cardiac Anesthesia, Department of Anesthesiology, Perioperative and Pain Medicine, Brigham and Women's Hospital, 75 Francis Street, Boston, MA 02115, USA; [b] Department of Anesthesiology, University of Tennessee College of Medicine, UTHSC/Regional One Health, Chandler Building, Suite 600, 877 Jefferson Avenue, Memphis, TN 38103, USA
* Corresponding author.
E-mail address: wgross@partners.org

Although there continues to be a place for sedative administration by trained nurses, nurse-administered moderate sedation is inadequate for procedures that require minimal patient movement or complex hemodynamic and respiratory control. The role of anesthesiologists in setting standards and determining the conditions for which moderate sedation is acceptable will advance the safety, efficiency, and quality of delivered care. As technological advancement continues, intricate techniques demand the full attention of proceduralists. Thus, the need for anesthesiology services beyond the operating room is escalating rapidly. Unfamiliar and unique work environments, new procedures, and moribund patients make expanded anesthesiology practice even more difficult yet more critical to accomplish.

Although this is a predictable consequence of medical evolution, strategic planning for the extension of anesthesiology services beyond the operating room has been slow to take shape. Because significant complications are relatively low-frequency events, complacency has prevailed. Muddled by misinformation, cultural barriers, poor communication, infrastructure deficits, and financial shortsightedness, the transition has been uneven and inefficient for patients, anesthesiologists, and proceduralists alike. Awareness of the need for collaborative, multidisciplinary financial, and medical planning is growing; the process is slow and difficult, however, because it involves intradisciplinary, multilevel infrastructure change, as well as cultural change among administrative and medical providers.

Disparities between operating room and nonoperating room practice standards are becoming increasingly obvious. Interventionalists and anesthesiologists alike are concerned. The Center for Medicare and Medicaid Studies (CMS), the Joint Commission (TJC), and the American Society of Anesthesiologists (ASA) all mandate preprocedural patient evaluation for high-risk patients and high-risk surgeries in the operating room.[4] Often, hospitals recognize and underwrite the cost of clinics that perform timely assessments of surgical patients. However, the provision of such services for interventional medicine patients, even as recommended by the ASA, is inconsistent at best. Clear pathways for financing those services are lacking, and medical guidelines for provision of such services are variable or nonexistent. Many hospitals seek to engage a broad base of primary cares providers by offering direct access scheduling; little if any preprocedural triage occurs. Assessments and workups are done immediately prior to the case, and planning does not occur. Comorbidities discovered at the last minute increase the likelihood of delays, cancellations, and suboptimal and excessively costly care.

In addition, inadequate screening leaves decisions about who needs an anesthesiologist undecided until immediately prior to the case. Scheduling becomes imprecise, and resources may not reflect need. Anesthesia providers and medical proceduralists are forced to wait for each other as a result of inaccurate scheduling, and overtime becomes necessary even when there is excess capacity during the day. Although the goal is for all scheduled operating room patients to undergo either a phone screen, a preoperative evaluation, or surgical contact prior to surgery, this is not always the case for patients scheduled for nonoperative procedures. Interventional medicine patients often present for their procedures having never seen the proceduralist and lacking any preoperative information.

Operating rooms generate significant revenue streams for hospitals, and they are expensive to maintain. Operating room management groups therefore prioritize efficient multidisciplinary function. Operating room utilization rates not only reflect the percentage of available time in use, but also the degree of practice integration that surgeons, anesthesiologists, and ancillary care providers achieve. In order to maximize utilization, central scheduling is utilized to coordinate operating room bookings and anesthesia resources. To minimize excess capacity, operating rooms are often closed when utilization falls below 70%.[5] No such management control exists for nonoperating room venues. Commonly, no hospital-wide group is responsible for consolidating, coordinating, or enforcing rules for scheduling elective nonoperating room cases, either within or between areas. Inconsistent scheduling prevails, and resource sharing is difficult. Lack of collaboratively organized scheduling leads to ineffective utilization of resources and equipment. Both anesthesiologists and interventionalists are left to juggle cases and personnel while attempting to define and integrate their own concepts of safety and efficiency across the medicine/surgery divide. Potential for outcome degradation and margin diminution increases.

Operational platforms throughout nonoperating room venues are inconsistent. In the operating room, stakeholders follow rules of collaborative practice in order to achieve common goals. Evaluation of patients prior to the day of surgery reduces medical errors, wasted resources, and unpredictability. Scheduling rules facilitate planning with respect to equipment, case process, booking flexibility, and pre- and postprocedure care. Improved utilization reduces cost and increases revenue. Similar hospital-based operational oversight of interventional medical venues is necessary, particularly in the context of increasing case volumes resulting from technological innovation and growing target populations. A central, multidisciplinary operational platform that coordinates the availability of anesthesiologists and the needs of interventional medicine providers across venues is needed. This may be an expensive undertaking, but it is a part of the hospital's cost of doing business just as it is in the operating room. Procedural suites scattered throughout hospitals, each operating according to its own rules, make consistent practice difficult; some centralization is essential. Surgeons and anesthesiologists are all too familiar with these problems in the operating room. If consistent high-quality care across surgical and interventional venues is to be provided, collaboration is necessary to provide a uniform hospital-based approach.[6,7] Variability and unpredictability are known to reduce efficiency. Missing patient evaluations cause delays and cancellations. Regular multidisciplinary oversight and consistent rules then emerged as a result of the need to accommodate more cases and to control costs. The parallels are clear: one ought not to make the same mistakes again.

Nonoperating room practice is a clear growth horizon for anesthesiologists, interventionalists, surgeons, and hospitals. Alignment of strategy and goals is needed here just as in the operating room. Success requires that nonoperating room areas function as multidisciplinary, strategic business units. Not all components of such units generate revenue, although they can be critical to that endpoint. A reframing of currently siloed departmental cost centers is called for.

From a patient care perspective, current disparities between operating room and interventional medicine procedural care are hard to defend. Why should a patient undergoing replacement of a stenotic heart valve, implantation of a ventricular assist device, excision of a cancerous colonic lesion, or treatment of a brain or lung tumor deserve a less rigorous or last-minute preprocedural evaluation, simply because the procedure is taking place in a procedural suite instead of an operating room, with an interventional medical provider instead of a surgeon? Efficiency depends upon effective planning that spans the episode of care from preoperative preparation to postoperative care. Why is the focus on efficiency within the operating room only, as operating room volumes remain flat, ignoring the inefficiency of nonoperating room procedures, as their numbers explode?

Hospital administrators have traditionally looked the other way when confronted with these questions, unaware of the impending medical and financial ramifications. As value-based care becomes more prevalent, it becomes clear that efficiency and outcome optimization are inter-related goals. One is impossible without the other. Inadequate patient preparation and idiosyncratic scheduling promotes inefficiency, poor patient progression, and increased length of stay. Decreased anesthesiology and proceduralist effectiveness diminishes hospital revenues by increasing uncompensated cost. Wait times for anesthesia-supported interventional case slots grow. As surgery and medicine move toward hybrid procedures, integrated care will demand hospital commitment to universal standards and collaborative platforms.

Anesthesiology sits at the fulcrum of care coordination. Interdisciplinary awareness, pre-emptive planning, and collaborative strategy design are essential components of patient-centric care. The physician's mission is to evaluate and safeguard patients through appropriate treatment, whatever the comorbidities of the patient, the exact nature of the treatment, and wherever that treatment occurs. Financial and medical norms of the future require a productive interface among anesthesiologists, surgeons, and interventional medicine providers.

REFERENCES

1. Gross WL, Weiss M. "Non OR Anesthesia". Chapter 90. In: Miller RD, Cohen NH, Eriksson LI, et al, editors. Miller's textbook of anesthesia. 8th edition. New York: Elsevier; 2014.
2. AHRQ HCUP Database.
3. Nagrebetsky A, Gabriel RA, Dutton RP, et al. Growth of nonoperating room anesthesia care in the United States: a contemporary trends analysis. Anesth Analg 2016. http://dx.doi.org/10.1213/ANE.0000000000001734.
4. US Code of Federal Regulations. §482.22(c) (5) and§482.24 (c) (1). Available at: http://www.cms.gov/Regulations-and-Guidance/Guidance/Manuals US Code of Federal Regulations. Accessed August 2, 2017.
5. Tyler DC, Pasquariello CA, Chen C. Determining optimum operating room utilization. Anesth Analg 2003;96:1114–21.
6. Correll DJ, Bader AM, Hull MW, et al. Value of preoperative clinic visits in identifying issues with potential impact on operating room efficiency. Anesthesiology 2006;105(6):1254–9 [discussion: 6A].
7. Marjamaa R, Vakkuri A, Kirvelä O. Operating room management: why, how and by whom? Acta Anaesthesiol Scand 2008;52(5):596–600.

Building and Maintaining Organizational Infrastructure to Attain Clinical Excellence

Kelly Lebak, MD[a], Jason Lane, MD, MPH[b], Richard Taus, MD[c],
Hansol Kim, MD[d,e], Michael S. Stecker, MD[d,e], Michael Hall, MD[f],
Meghan B. Lane-Fall, MD, MSHP[g], Mark S. Weiss, MD[f,*]

KEYWORDS

- Interdisciplinary/multidisciplinary • Protocols • Standardization • Closed claims
- Curriculum • Quality metrics • Safety • Adverse event

KEY POINTS

- This article describes the considerations for building an organizational infrastructure dedicated to the care of patients undergoing procedures requiring anesthesia services outside the traditional operating room.
- This article brings into focus how to build a leadership team and standardized work environment necessary for the safe and effective provision of non–operating room anesthesia (NORA).
- This article introduces a new paradigm for education of anesthesiology trainees focusing on NORA.
- This article elaborates on the requirements for a robust system of quality assurance and improvement focused on the unique challenges presented by NORA.

[a] Case Western Reserve University School of Medicine, MetroHealth Medical Center, Brecksville Ambulatory Surgery Center, Cleveland, OH 44109, USA; [b] Department of Anesthesiology, Vanderbilt University Medical Center, 1301 Medical Center Drive, 4648 TVC, Nashville, TN 37232, USA; [c] SMG Radiology, Morton Hospital, 88 Washington Street, Taunton, MA 02780, USA; [d] Division of Angiography and Interventional Radiology, Department of Radiology, Brigham and Women's Hospital, 75 Francis Street, Midcampus SR-340, Boston, MA 02115, USA; [e] Harvard Medical School, 25 Shattuck Street Boston, MA 02115, USA; [f] Department of Anesthesiology and Critical Care, Hospital of the University of Pennsylvania, 3400 Spruce Street, 6th Floor Dulles Building, Philadelphia, PA 19104, USA; [g] Department of Anesthesiology and Critical Care, University of Pennsylvania Perelman School of Medicine, 309 Blockley Hall, 423 Guardian Drive, Philadelphia, PA 19104, USA
* Corresponding author.
E-mail addresses: Mark.Weiss@uphs.upenn.edu; weissm@uphs.upenn.edu

Anesthesiology Clin 35 (2017) 559–568
http://dx.doi.org/10.1016/j.anclin.2017.07.002

Modern medicine increasingly distinguishes itself from historical practice in that it depends heavily on collaboration between teams that are both interdisciplinary and interprofessional. The National Academy of Medicine, formerly the Institute of Medicine, recommends interdisciplinary team training to enhance patient safety and the quality of health care.[1] To attain clinical excellence in any realm of medicine, the importance of teams must be reinforced, and resources should be devoted to creation and ongoing support of these teams. Once created, an effective team can establish and implement standards for both patients and the shared work environment. This approach has been well recognized in the ICU to improve outcomes for critically ill patients.[2] Once standards and protocols are established, quality assurance and improvement processes must be enacted to ensure the protocols are patient centered and applied appropriately. Appropriate patient care may require deviation from a given protocol; resilient teams are able to work together to make decisions about when to adjust protocols.[3] This interdisciplinary team approach with structured quality improvement and assurance has been enacted in many areas of medicine since the National Academy of Medicine published its landmark article, "To Err Is Human,"[1] and it is increasingly applied to non–operating room anesthesia (NORA).

This article describes considerations for building an organizational infrastructure dedicated to the care of patients undergoing procedures requiring anesthesia services outside the traditional operating room. First, building a leadership team and standardized work environment necessary for the safe and effective provision of NORA is discussed and then a new paradigm for education of anesthesiology trainees focusing on NORA is laid out. Finally, the requirements for a robust system of quality assurance and improvement focused on the unique challenges presented by NORA are elaborated.

ESTABLISHING COMPREHENSIVE TEAMS

Medical proceduralists, including interventional radiologists, gastroenterologists, and electrophysiologists, have similar expectations for patients undergoing diagnostic or therapeutic procedures. Proceduralists want patients to be safe and comfortable during the procedure while achieving conditions (eg, lack of movement) adequate for performing a procedure. To provide comfort while minimizing the untoward effects of sedative agents, proceduralists frequently use local anesthetics. Moderate sedation may be used when procedures are too stimulating for local anesthetics alone or when a patient is too anxious or otherwise unable to tolerate the procedure while fully alert. Preprocedural evaluation by the procedural team helps distinguish patient cases appropriate for minimal or moderate sedation from those who may require deep sedation or general anesthesia.

There are multiple drug classes that proceduralists may use as sedatives, such as anxiolytics (eg, midazolam) and opioids (eg, fentanyl). During sedation supervised by proceduralists (as opposed to sedation administered by an anesthesia team), a separate trained staff member, typically a nurse, monitors the patient and administers the sedating medications. Ultimately the proceduralist remains responsible for medication doses and for monitoring a patient's vital signs during the administration of sedative medications.

The task of sedation necessarily draws an operator's attention away from the procedure. This may lengthen the procedure and increase risk to the patient. Provision of sedation by anesthesia staff allows proceduralists to concentrate on the intervention without distraction, but it is impractical for anesthesia staff to be involved in the care of every patient undergoing minimally invasive procedures. The factors that have an impact on provision of anesthesia services within the NORA suite include limited staff availability, increased time required for initiation of and recovery from sedation, anesthesia staff comfort with NORA suite equipment, and anesthesia staff familiarity with minimally invasive procedures. Using radiology as an example, anesthesiologists accustomed to caring for patients in operating rooms with standard configurations may encounter difficulty caring for patients requiring radiology procedures. Radiologists often have several different suites in which procedures may be performed: fluoroscopy, CT, MRI, PET, and ultrasound. Although ultrasound may be mobile, even available in a traditional operating room, the other modalities are not portable, and the selection of a diagnostic or therapeutic modality is not usually negotiable. The radiology suites may not have been designed with anesthesia services in mind and may have limited space. Although oxygen and suction are likely available, a data drop and gas scavenger system may not be. An anesthesiologist should become familiar with the capabilities and limitations of each suite. It has become commonplace for new suites to include an anesthesiologist in the planning phase, but older suites will remain in use for years to come.

Anesthesiologists should also become familiar with the demands of the particular procedure. As an example, most radiologists request anesthesia assistance during creation of a transjugular intrahepatic portosystemic shunt.[4] Patients undergoing this procedure often have cirrhosis and portal hypertension, and the procedure may be elective or emergent. Although the operator and sterile field are probably at the right neck, the procedure is in the liver. Monitoring devices or cables overlying the abdomen are not acceptable. When the shunt is created, the large volume of blood suddenly returning to the right atrium may cause hemodynamic instability. In the electrophysiology laboratory, patients with a proclivity for potentially fatal arrhythmias must be managed through long interventions that may themselves induce dangerous arrhythmias or otherwise put patients at risk for several serious complications.[5] To effectively manage a patient undergoing such procedures, an anesthesiologist must be knowledgeable about the procedure as well as the patient and must maintain open communication with the interventionalist throughout the course of the procedure.[5,6]

Ideally, a multidisciplinary leadership team that includes proceduralists, anesthesiologists, nurses, and support staff would collaborate to decide which patients and procedures require the provision of anesthesia care. There are logistical barriers to forming the multidisciplinary leadership team necessary to provide safe and efficient patient care in the NORA suite. First, it is important to identify personnel who are both willing and able to work across disciplines to promote safe NORA care. Specifically, leaders from each discipline (ie, proceduralists, anesthesia, nursing, and support services) should demonstrate an interest in developing common goals and in working together to achieve them. Second, guidelines are necessary to facilitate the determination of which patients are likely to need anesthesia services. In one study, most institutions did not have explicit guidelines for which procedures should use anesthesia services, even though a majority of respondents believed such guidelines improve patient care.[4] Third, lack of universal availability of anesthesia staff may limit the ability to provide anesthesia services when requested. In a recently published survey of interventional radiologists, approximately half of respondents believed anesthesia support during off-hours and on weekends was inadequate, especially for emergent cases (differentiated from elective, scheduled cases occurring during off-hours).[4]

As discussed previously, effective utilization of time and provider availability are major concerns and perceived as problems by interventionalists considering the use of anesthesia services. Although many interventional procedures are performed urgently on unscheduled patients, many can be scheduled with anesthesiology and with time for a thorough preanesthesia evaluation. In departments with a sufficient volume of cases, there can be regularly scheduled blocks of time with anesthesiology. It is reasonable to assume that more frequent participation by designated anesthesiologists will lead to some greater efficiency of time as well as a building of trust between the 2 disciplines during the management of medically complex patients undergoing invasive procedures away from the operating room.

STANDARDS FOR THE WORK ENVIRONMENT

Regardless of the location or type of anesthesia that is administered, the American Society of Anesthesiologists (ASA) has set minimum standards for physiologic monitoring that include oxygenation, ventilation, circulation, and temperature as well as the presence of qualified anesthesia personnel for the duration of all anesthetics.[7] Additionally, the ASA has published further guidelines NORA that should be followed unless for some reason "they are not applicable to the individual patient or care setting."[8] These guidelines are as follows:

1. A source of oxygen, preferably piped in, with a backup supply
2. A source of suction that preferably meets operating room standards
3. A scavenging system if inhalational anesthetics are used
4. ASA basic monitoring, a hand resuscitator bag, anesthesia drugs and equipment, and, if using inhalation anesthesia, an anesthesia machine maintained to operating room standards
5. An adequate number of electrical outlets for all anesthesia equipment with isolated electric power or ground fault circuit interrupters if in a wet location (eg, cystoscopy, arthroscopy, or labor and delivery birthing room)[9]
6. Adequate lighting of the patient and anesthesia equipment plus a form of light that is battery operated that is not a laryngoscope
7. Adequate space for all equipment and personnel to allow easy access to the patient
8. Emergency equipment, including a defibrillator and medications
9. Adequate staff capable of supporting the anesthesiologist and 2-way communication to call for help
10. Observation of all building and safety codes and facility standards
11. Appropriate postanesthesia care, including personnel and equipment

According to the ASA, sedation is a continuum, with minimal sedation at one end and general anesthesia at the other.[10] Often, proceduralists without specific training in anesthesiology direct the administration of medications to induce and maintain minimal or moderate sedation to facilitate the performance of a procedure. Minimal sedation is considered equivalent to anxiolysis, and the patient maintains a normal response to verbal stimulation and commands. Airway reflexes, ventilation, and cardiovascular status are not affected. With moderate sedation, the patient still has a purposeful reaction to verbal or light touch stimulation, and airway, ventilation, and cardiovascular status is maintained without interventions. Deep sedation is achieved when a patient is not easily aroused to voice or light touch but does have a purposeful reaction to repeated or painful stimulation. As with general anesthesia, the airway and ventilation may need to be supported, yet cardiovascular function is usually stable. Lastly, when under general anesthesia, the patient is unarousable even with painful stimulation, and the airway, ventilation, and cardiovascular function often need to be supported.[10] When interventionalists request monitored anesthesia care (MAC) as the anesthesia type for a procedure, what is often meant is deep sedation or general anesthesia without the use of an airway device (endotracheal tube or laryngeal mask). They likely do not realize that MAC has been defined by the ASA to include the "anesthesia assessment and management of a patient's actual or anticipated physiologic derangements or medical problems that may occur during a diagnostic or therapeutic procedure"[11] and "sedatives, analgesics, hypnotics, anesthetic agents or other medications"[12] may or may not be given. In practice, however, rarely is MAC provided without administering any medications.

In an analysis from the ASA closed claims database, 50% of the claims that were identified as taking place in a remote location involved MAC.[13] There was a significantly greater proportion of death in remote locations, with respiratory complications (in particular inadequate oxygenation/ventilation) more common than in the claims related to operating room care. More claims involving remote locations versus operating rooms were deemed to have been preventable by using better monitoring. Given increasing volume of non–operating room cases for anesthesiologists, these increased risks must be acknowledged and addressed.

The most recent ASA "Standards for Basic Anesthetic Monitoring" states that in regard to ventilation, only qualitative clinical signs need to be monitored during regional and local anesthesia as long as no sedation is given.[7] The ASA specifically states that during moderate or deep sedation, in addition to qualitative signs of ventilation, the "presence" of exhaled carbon dioxide (CO_2) should be monitored continually.[7] This is most commonly done using capnometry, which is the quantitative measurement of exhaled CO_2, along with a graphic display of the measured CO_2 versus time (capnography).[14] Although these monitors are accurate when attached to an advanced airway device, when used with a nasal cannula there likely is dilution of exhaled gases with air and oxygen because it is not a closed system; capnometry values measures lower than the true end-tidal CO_2. What is most useful is identification of changes in the shape of the capnogram, respiratory rate, and deviation from baseline values (ie, prior to any sedation).[15]

There is varying evidence on the benefit of capnography in preventing hypoxemia during sedation cases. In a 2011 meta-analysis, respiratory complications (depressions, apneas, desaturations, obstructions, and need for supplemental oxygen) were 17.6 times more likely to be detected if capnography was used along with standard monitoring during sedation cases.[16] In a 2016 meta-analysis,[17] capnography decreased hypoxic episodes but did not decrease the need for assisted ventilation. Additionally, this finding was only true when propofol was used for sedation during colonoscopies. Due to the risks of bias and heterogeneity, this evidence was considered poor quality.[17] Despite the paucity of strong, evidence-based data to support the use of capnography to reduce hypoxemia and its sequelae, the authors consider its use to be the best practice for monitoring ventilation in a sedated patient with a natural airway. This is particularly true in NORA sites where a patient may not be fully accessible or visible to anesthesiology personnel. It is the duty of leaders in patient safety to model the use of standardized practice parameters to minimize patient risk; this should begin with the application of the ASA long-standing standards regarding basic monitors.

TEACHING CLINICAL EXCELLENCE

Effective patient-care teams require members skilled in their own fields and knowledgeable about the attributes and skill sets of the other members of the team. To create active and effective members of these interprofessional and interdisciplinary clinical teams, anesthesiology training programs must prepare trainees for the unique challenges of providing anesthesia care in the non–operating room setting. Providers accustomed to the traditional operating room may be uncomfortable in non–operating room sites that are more often lacking in space, equipment, or access to medications. Non–operating room locations may be far from operating room support, and obtaining assistance from anesthesia colleagues may prove challenging.[18] There is a trend toward performing more complex procedures for patients with higher acuity of illness in these environments. The expansion of NORA in both volume and complexity, however, has not correlated with an increase in exposure to NORA for anesthesiology trainees (**Fig. 1**).[19]

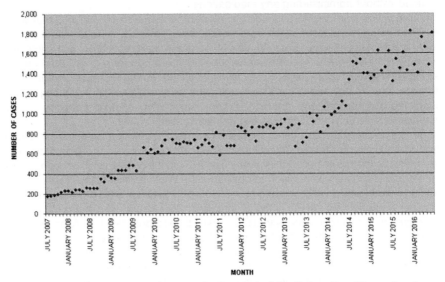

Fig. 1. Growth of NORA case volume at the Hospital of the University of Pennsylvania.

Until recently, formal training in this subspecialty of anesthesia has been modest. In 2006, Hausman and colleagues[19] distributed a 14-question survey to the 134 listed members of the Society of Academic Anesthesia Chairs and the Association of Anesthesiology Program Directors to better understand the clinical exposure of anesthesiology residents to NORA. Survey respondents reported that residents had minimal exposure to anesthesia in the non–operating room setting, and approximately half of anesthesiology residency programs offered no office-based anesthesia experience.

Since the Hausman survey, there has been explosive growth of NORA cases performed (**Fig. 2**), in both number and variety, across multiple subspecialties of medicine. NORA cases now comprise approximately one-third of the cases reported to the National Anesthesia Clinical Outcomes Registry. Research using National

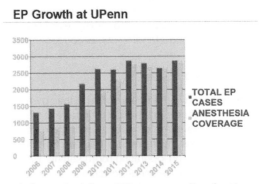

Fig. 2. Growth of total electrophysiology (EP) cases as well as fraction requiring anesthesia services at the Hospital of the University of Pennsylvania (UPenn).

Anesthesia Clinical Outcomes Registry data demonstrates that NORA is a rapidly growing component of overall anesthesia practice.[20] This growth is linked to both technological advancement reducing the need for invasive surgeries, and the aging and rising comorbidity of the population, increasing overall health care consumption.

In July 2016, the Accreditation Council for Graduate Medical Education (ACGME)[21] formally addressed the deficit defined by Hausman and colleagues,[19] by requiring that anesthesiology residents have at least 2 weeks of experience managing the anesthetic care of patients undergoing diagnostic or therapeutic procedures outside the surgical suite. This new requirement offers both the opportunity and the challenge to create a comprehensive curriculum for NORA education. Although the type and location of these cases are not specified, a well-rounded curriculum (including hands-on experience/reading materials/didactic interaction/Web-based self-guided learning) that features a broad exposure to many types of procedures would be optimal. Not only has the push to improve the ability of the anesthesia workforce to manage patients in the NORA realm come from the ACGME but also NORA-specific education has been undertaken by the ASA with dedicated NORA CME.

To address the NORA requirements of the ACGME, the Department of Anesthesiology and Critical Care at the University of Pennsylvania created and developed a 2-week NORA rotation meant to familiarize residents with challenging cases involving high-acuity patients. This rotation is supplemented by an extensive, Web-based curriculum (NORAlink.org), including NORA-specific literature, lectures, and problem-based learning modules.[22] Although implementation strategies vary, the utilization of Web-based learning continues to increase in medical training, and NORAlink.org is designed to complement the clinical learning of residents outside the time and attention constraints of the procedure suite.[23–25]

QUALITY IMPROVEMENT

To attain clinical excellence consistent with the modern era of health care reform, NORA providers must embrace a culture of quality improvement and focus on providing value-based care. Anesthesiology, as a specialty, has already emerged as a leader in quality and safety.[1] In recent years, however, anesthetics administered in non–operating room settings have been linked to several high-profile deaths, increasing public concern for the safety of anesthesia outside the operating room.[26]

Leadership Commitment to Quality Improvement

Fostering a culture within any practice group that encourages and supports quality improvement activities requires a commitment from departmental leadership. This includes the designation of specific individuals within a department to act as leaders and facilitators of quality improvement initiatives. In any department with specific resources dedicated to NORA, a quality improvement officer can be specifically focused on NORA given the unique opportunities for quality improvement NORA presents. Importantly, by focusing individual efforts on NORA, teams of key stakeholders in the NORA clinical space can be developed, including, but not limited to, anesthesiologists, proceduralists, certified registered nurse anesthetists (CRNAs), trainees, and support staff. An interdisciplinary approach to solving clinical problems is paramount to effect change and improve patient outcomes.

Many clinical academic departments have quality improvement committees; however, these are often focused on reviewing patient safety events and leading morbidity and mortality conferences. Committees may not have the resources or structure to effectively implement quality improvement initiatives.[27]

Physician training organizations have recognized the importance of creating leaders in the quality and safety domains. The ACGME has identified knowledge of patient safety and quality improvement as core competencies expected of anesthesia residents. In the ACGME Anesthesiology Milestones Project of 2014, 2 of the 25 milestones on which residents are evaluated are "Patient Safety and Quality Improvement" and "Incorporation of Quality Improvement and Patient Safety Initiatives into Personal Practice."[28]

Safety Reporting

A characteristic of high reliability organizations is having a nonpunitive system for reporting adverse events to identify safety and quality issues. In medicine, preventable adverse outcomes came to light with the Institute of Medicine's publication of "To Err Is Human," which concluded that more than 1 million preventable adverse events occurred in the United States each year, of which an estimated 44,000 to 98,000 resulted in patient mortality.[1] In the interest of reducing preventable harm, many institutions have implemented voluntary event reporting systems for reporting patient safety events. The purpose of these systems is to identify events resulting in harm to patients as well as near misses, which are unsafe conditions that did not result in harm but that could have caused harm had the error not been identified. Any error or near miss identified by an anesthesia provider in the non–operating room environment would be entered within this system.

There are several challenges when it comes to implementing adverse event reporting, the most prominent being the fear of repercussion by the individual identifying the event.[29] To ensure effective identification of adverse events and potentially unsafe conditions, the organization must develop a culture in which event reporting is viewed solely as an opportunity to identify opportunities for improvement and not as a mechanism for assigning blame or liability. Other challenges include decreasing barriers to event reporting by ensuring the reporting system is user friendly and not overly time consuming. Furthermore, a dedicated team should review these events regularly, and opportunities for improvement should be identified and acted on through a structured process. To achieve clinical excellence in the NORA space, it is essential to rapidly identify patient safety events through adverse outcome reporting, allowing for interventions that improve clinical practice and patient safety.

Using Data: Electronic Medical Records and Dashboards

Both governmental agencies and insurance agencies are increasingly requiring public reporting of patient safety and outcome metrics for practice comparison and for determining compensation. The first initiative to measure hospital quality began in 1998 with the Joint Commission ORYX program. At this time, hospitals were required to report performance measures using nonstandardized data.[30] The Centers for Medicare and Medicaid Services now requires the collection of more than 50 inpatient measures with more than 30 of these measures publicly reported.[31]

The wide availability of electronic medical records lends itself to the automated abstraction of data for quality improvement. The challenge is choosing appropriate process and outcome metrics that accurately characterize current practice and subsequently reflect meaningful changes over time in response to the implementation of quality improvement projects. Pain score, for example, is a subjective metric that may not accurately capture a successful pain reduction intervention. Instead, measuring total postoperative opioid consumption or the need for breakthrough pain medication doses might be a preferred method to address this question.

Quality metrics are used not only at the national and organization levels but also at the level of individual clinicians. Clinician-specific dashboards are increasingly developed to provide feedback to anesthesiologists regarding their practice. These can be used to identify outliers to help change individual and group practice as well as drive quality improvement. If dashboards are developed using reliable metrics and implemented in a nonpunitive manner, they can be powerful tools to measure variability in practice, identify opportunities for change, and track impact of quality interventions.

SUMMARY

Active maintenance of highly functional teams is critical to ensuring safe, efficient patient care in the NORA suite. In addition to developing collaborative relationships and patient care protocols, individual and team training is needed. For anesthesiologists, this training must begin during residency, and the ACGME has recently acted to ensure all anesthesiology residents receive NORA-specific training. This training should be supplemented with continuing education in this field for providers who find themselves working in the NORA space, and NORAlink.org has been created to fill this need. As NORA continues to grow, robust, NORA-specific quality assurance and improvement programs will empower anesthesiologists with the tools they need to best care for our patients.

REFERENCES

1. Kohn LT, Corrigan JM, Molla S. To err is human. Medicine (Baltimore) 1999;126: 312.
2. Pronovost PJ, Angus DC, Dorman T, et al. Physician staffing patterns and clinical outcomes in critically ill patients: a systematic review. JAMA 2002;288(17): 2151–62.
3. Girbes ARJ, Robert R, Marik PE. Protocols: help for improvement but beware of regression to the mean and mediocrity. Intensive Care Med 2015;41(12): 2218–20.
4. Natcheva HN, Silberzweig JE, Chao CP, et al. Survey of current status and physician opinion regarding ancillary staffing for the IR suite. J Vasc Interv Radiol 2014; 25(11):1777–84.
5. Kwak J. Anesthesia for electrophysiology studies and catheter ablations. Semin Cardiothorac Vasc Anesth 2013;17(3):195–202.
6. Price A, Santucci P. Electrophysiology procedures: weighing the factors affecting choice of anesthesia. Semin Cardiothorac Vasc Anesth 2013;17(3):203–11.
7. American Society of Anesthesiologists, editor. Standards for basic anesthetic monitoring. Park Ridge (IL): American Society of Anesthesiologists; 2015.
8. American Society of Anesthesiologists, editor. Statement on nonoperating room anesthetizing locations. Park Ridge (IL): American Society of Anesthesiologists; 2013.
9. National Fire Protection Association, editor. NFPA 99: standard for health care facilities. Quincy (MA): National Fire Protection Association (NFPA); 2015.
10. American Society of Anesthesiologists, editor. Continuum of depth of sedation: definition of general anesthesia and levels of sedation/analgesia. Park Ridge (IL): American Society of Anesthesiologists; 2014.
11. American Society of Anesthesiologists, editor. Distinguishing monitored anesthesia care ("MAC") from moderate sedation/analgesia (conscious sedation). Park Ridge (IL): American Society of Anesthesiologists; 2013.

12. American Society of Anesthesiologists, editor. Position on monitored anesthesia care. Park Ridge, IL: American Society of Anesthesiologists; 2013.
13. Metzner J, Posner KL, Domino KB. The risk and safety of anesthesia at remote locations: the US closed claims analysis. Curr Opin Anaesthesiol 2009;22(4): 502–8.
14. Siobal MS. Monitoring exhaled carbon dioxide. Respir Care 2016;61(10): 1397–416.
15. Kodali BS. Capnography outside the operating rooms. Anesthesiology 2013; 118(1):192–201.
16. Waugh JB, Epps CA, Khodneva YA. Capnography enhances surveillance of respiratory events during procedural sedation: a meta-analysis. J Clin Anesth 2011; 23(3):189–96.
17. Conway A, Douglas C, Sutherland JR. A systematic review of capnography for sedation. Anaesthesia 2016;71(4):450–4.
18. Chang B, Urman RD. Non-operating Room Anesthesia. The principles of patient assessment and preparation. Anesthesiol Clin 2016;34(1):223–40.
19. Hausman LM, Levine AI, Rosenblatt MA. A survey evaluating the training of anesthesiology residents in office-based anesthesia. J Clin Anesth 2006;18(7): 499–503.
20. Nagrebetsky A, Gabriel RA, Dutton RP, et al. Growth of nonoperating room anesthesia care in the United States: a contemporary trends analysis. Anesth Analg 2017;124(4):1261–7.
21. Accreditation Council for Graduate Medical Education, editor. ACGME program requirements for graduate medical education in anesthesiology. Chicago: Accreditation Council for Graduate Medical Education; 2016.
22. Weiss M. NORAlink. Available at: http://www.noralink.org.2017.
23. Close A, Goldberg A, Helenowski I, et al. Beta test of web-based virtual patient decision-making exercises for residents demonstrates discriminant validity and learning. J Surg Educ 2015;72(6):e130–6.
24. Lakshmanan A, Leeman KT, Brodsky D, et al. Evaluation of a web-based portal to improve resident education by neonatology fellows. Med Educ Online 2014; 19:24403.
25. Hindle A, Cheng J, Thabane L, et al. Web-based learning for emergency airway management in anesthesia residency training. Anesthesiol Res Pract 2015;2015. http://dx.doi.org/10.1155/2015/971406.
26. Rice S. Joan Rivers' death highlights risks in outpatient surgery for seniors. Mod Healthc 2014;44(37):11.
27. Boudreaux AM, Vetter TR. The creation and impact of a dedicated section on quality and patient safety in a clinical academic department. Acad Med 2013; 88(2):173–8.
28. The anesthesiology milestone project. J Grad Med Educ 2014;6(1 Suppl 1): 15–28.
29. Leape LL. Reporting of adverse events. N Engl J Med 2002;347(20):1633–8.
30. Lee KY, Loeb JM, Nadzam DM, et al. An overview of the joint commission's ORYX initiative and proposed statistical methods. Heal Serv Outcomes Res Methodol 2000;1(1):63–73.
31. Chassin MR, Loeb JM, Schmaltz SP, et al. Accountability measures–using measurement to promote quality improvement. N Engl J Med 2010;363(7):683–8.

Safety of Non–Operating Room Anesthesia

A Closed Claims Update

Zachary G. Woodward, MD[a],
Richard D. Urman, MD, MBA, FASA[a,b],*, Karen B. Domino, MD, MPH[c]

KEYWORDS

- Closed claims • Non–operating room anesthesia (NORA) • Remote anesthesia
- Gastroenterology • Cardiology • Radiology • Sedation • Medical malpractice

KEY POINTS

- Malpractice claims for non–operating room anesthesia care (NORA) had a higher proportion of claims for death compared with operating room (OR) settings.
- Aspiration pneumonitis occurred in a higher proportion of NORA malpractice claims, compared with claims in OR settings.
- NORA claims most frequently involved monitored anesthesia care. Inadequate oxygenation/ventilation was responsible for nearly one-third of NORA claims.
- Malpractice claims for NORA were less frequent than claims for OR anesthesia as assessed by the number of anesthetics in NORA versus OR locations.
- NORA claims occurred more frequently in cardiology and radiology locations compared with the number of anesthetics in these procedural locations, suggesting a higher risk of adverse events in these locations.

INTRODUCTION

Providing anesthesia services in non–operating room (OR) settings is a rapidly changing and growing challenge. As technologies advance and the financial landscape of health care continues to transform, many of the novel therapies and

Disclosure Statement: The authors have no financial interests to disclose. The Anesthesia Closed Claims project and National Anesthesia Clinical Outcome Registry are funded by the Anesthesia Quality Institute. Richard D. Urman: Member, AQI Data Use Committee; Funding from Medtronic for unrelated research.

[a] Department of Anesthesiology, Perioperative and Pain Medicine, Brigham and Women's Hospital, 75 Francis Street, Boston, MA 02115, USA; [b] Center for Perioperative Research, Brigham and Women's Hospital, Boston, MA 02115, USA; [c] Department of Anesthesiology and Pain Medicine, University of Washington, 1959 Northeast Pacific Street, Box 356540, Seattle, WA 98195, USA
* Corresponding author. Department of Anesthesiology, Perioperative and Pain Medicine, Brigham and Women's Hospital, 75 Francis Street, Boston, MA 02115.
E-mail address: rurman@bwh.harvard.edu

treatments being integrated into practice are now performed outside of the traditional OR. Increasingly complex procedures are calling for more invasive monitoring, deeper sedation, and a higher rate of general anesthesia.[1,2] The patient population is also increasing in age and disease burden as anesthesiologists are more frequently caring for patients with multiple comorbidities in unfamiliar locations.[3] Although the proportion of remote site anesthesia cases continues to increase, the risks and the rates of adverse outcomes in non–OR anesthesia (NORA) are poorly defined when compared with the OR setting.[4] Older analyses of closed malpractice claims suggested an increased risk of NORA compared with the OR setting.[5,6] Because procedures, patients, regulatory requirements, and anesthesia practice have changed considerably, we reviewed remote location anesthesia claims using the Anesthesia Closed Claims database for injuries occurring between 2000 and 2012 and compared them with claims from anesthesia care for OR procedures. In addition, we evaluated current trends and outcomes in NORA using data from the National Anesthesia Clinical Outcomes Registry (NACOR) and compared them with NORA closed claims.

METHODS
Closed Claims Project Methodology

The Anesthesia Closed Claims Project database is a structured collection of closed anesthesia malpractice claims described in detail elsewhere.[7,8] Briefly, on-site anesthesiologist–reviewers abstracted data from closed anesthesia malpractice claims onto detailed data collection instruments at participating professional liability companies across the United States. The panel of 22 companies (at the time of this report) insured approximately one-third of practicing anesthesiologists in the United States. Information was collected from medical records, consultant evaluations, expert witness reports, claims manager summaries, and legal summaries. Data collected included patient demographics, type of surgery, details regarding anesthesia care, patient outcomes, and legal outcomes. The on-site reviewer evaluated the outcome, severity of injury, and cause of injury (ie, damaging event), and summarized the claim in a brief narrative, including the sequence of events and causes of injury. The Closed Claims Project Investigator Committee reviewed the claims, and any disagreements in assessments were resolved by committee members.

For this report, we used the Anesthesia Closed Claims Project database of 10,357 claims. Inclusion criteria were claims associated with surgical or procedural anesthesia care. Claims associated with obstetric anesthesia (including cesarean section) and those associated with acute or chronic pain medicine were not included. NORA location claims were further reviewed to assess how sedation contributed to the primary damaging event. In-depth analysis was performed on NORA claims in which absolute or relative oversedation during the procedure precipitated the series of events leading to injury. Claims for the current report involved events that occurred from 2000 to 2012, of which 1900 were in OR or NORA locations.

NACOR data were provided by the Anesthesia Quality Institute (AQI) and adapted from Chang and colleagues.[9] NACOR is a large registry that collects electronic reports of anesthesia care in the United States. Reporting is voluntary and the AQI estimated that, in 2015, NACOR included 25% of all United States anesthesia cases.[10] The location of cases is listed for the majority of records, making categorization to OR and NORA possible. The NACOR dataset used 12,252,846 total cases, of which 9,890,875 were OR or NORA cases from January 1, 2010, to December 31, 2013. Cases for obstetric procedures and records without location data were excluded.

For the figures comparing closed claims with NACOR, the NACOR data were analyzed and recalculated to fit the definitions in closed claims to allow comparison with closed claims data.

Statistical Analysis

For closed claims, NORA claims were compared with OR claims. All payments made to the plaintiff were extracted from the database and adjusted to 2016 dollar amounts with the Consumer Price Index.[11] Median and interquartile ranges were reported for payments because they were not normally distributed. Claims with no payment were excluded from calculation of median and interquartile range. Proportions were compared using Fisher's exact test, t-test for equality of means (age), or Mann-Whitney U test (payment amount). All statistical analysis used SPSS 22 for Windows (IBM Corporation, Armonk, NY) with $P<.05$ as the criterion for statistical significance and 2-tailed tests.

RESULTS

Out of 1900 closed claims for injuries from 2000 to 2012, 72 involved procedures in NORA locations compared with 1828 claims involving procedures within the OR. The NACOR dataset consisted of 9,890,875 NACOR cases from 2010 to 2013, with 1,900,043 NORA cases.

Patient and Case Characteristics

NORA claims were more likely to involve a patient under the age of 16 (10% <16 years of age; $P<.05$) than OR claims (**Table 1**). Patients in NORA claims were more likely to be an American Society of Anesthesiologists (ASA) physical status score of 3 to 5 compared with OR claims (66% vs 51%; $P<.01$). Monitored anesthesia care (MAC) was the predominant anesthetic technique for NORA claims (69% of claims, compared with only 9% in OR claims; see **Table 1**; $P<.01$).

Non–Operating Room Anesthesia Care Claims by Specific Location and Anesthetic Technique

Most of the NORA claims occurred in the gastrointestinal (GI) suite (51%) and 89% were MAC cases (**Table 2**). The next 2 most common locations were the cardiology catheterization and electrophysiology laboratories (29% of NORA claims) and the radiology suite (17% of NORA claims). Both of these locations involved MAC less frequently at 57% and 33%, respectively (see **Table 2**).

Common Complications and Severity of Injuries

The proportion of claims for death in NORA claims was more than twice that of OR claims (**Table 3** and **Fig. 1**; 61% vs 30%; $P<.001$). The proportion of temporary or non-disabling injuries was increased in OR claims compared with NORA claims, whereas permanent disabling injuries were represented in similar proportions for NORA and OR claims (see **Fig. 1**). Aspiration pneumonitis occurred more frequently ($P<.01$) and nerve injury less frequently ($P<.001$) in NORA claims than in OR claims (see **Table 3**).

Mechanisms of Injury

The proportion of adverse respiratory events in NORA was more than twice that of OR claims (**Table 4**; 53% vs 23%; $P<.001$). Inadequate oxygenation/ventilation was the most common respiratory-related injury in NORA claims and was increased compared with OR claims (**Fig. 2**; 31% vs 6%; $P<.001$). Other respiratory-related NORA claims

Table 1
Patient and case characteristics and liability in NORA claims versus OR claims

	NORA Claims (N = 72), n (%)	OR Claims (N = 1828), n (%)	P Value
Age (y) (n = 1878)			
Mean age ± SD	50.9 ± 21.0	50.4 ± 18.1	.874
>70 y (n = 1878)	10 (14)	262 (14)	.565
<16 y	7 (10)	77 (4)	.037
Sex (n = 1898)			.115
Female	32 (45)	969 (53)	
Male	39 (55)	858 (47)	
ASA physical status (n = 1853)			.007
1–2	24 (34)	880 (49)	
3–5	47 (66)	902 (51)	
Procedure status (n = 1878)			.201
Emergent	11 (15)	209 (12)	
Elective	60 (85)	1598 (88)	
Primary anesthetic technique (n = 1897)			<.001
MAC	50 (69)	168 (9)	
GA	17 (24)	1327 (73)	
Regional	1 (1)	189 (10)	
Both GA and regional	0 (0)	118 (6)	
None	4 (6)	23 (1)	
Liability characteristics			
Substandard care (n = 1697)	42 (66)	714 (44)	<.001
Preventable by better monitoring (n = 1773)	23 (35)	290 (17)	<.001
Payment made ($) (n = 1885)	52 (72)	1038 (57)	.007
Median payment ($) (2016$)	$571,109	$294,323	.004
25% quartile	$268,998	$94,734	
75% quartile	$1,295,225	$858,866	

N = 1900 claims unless otherwise stated.

Payments adjusted to 2016 dollar amounts using Consumer Price Index. Claims with missing information were excluded. Claims with no payment excluded from median/interquartile range.

Abbreviations: ASA, American Society of Anesthesiologists; GA, general anesthesia; MAC, monitored anesthesia care; NORA, non–operating room anesthesia; OR, operating room; SD, standard deviation.

included aspiration of gastric contents (11%), difficult intubation (7%), and esophageal intubation (7%). NORA claims related to regional anesthesia were less frequent than in OR claims (P<.001; see **Table 4**). Other damaging events such as cardiovascular (14%), medication (6%), and equipment-related events did not differ significantly between claims arising from the 2 locations (see **Table 4**).

Characteristics of Non–Operating Room Anesthesia Care Claims Associated with Oversedation

Oversedation leading to respiratory depression was judged to be responsible for 20 NORA claims, with two-thirds occuring in the GI suite (**Table 5**). Propofol was the

Table 2
NORA claims by location and anesthetic technique (n = 72)

Location	Claims n (%)	MAC, n (% of Location Group)	GA, n (% of Location Group)
Gastrointestinal suite	37 (51)	33 (89)	4 (11)
Cardiology	21 (29)	12 (57)	7 (33)
Radiology	12 (17)	4 (33)	6 (50)
Lithotripsy	2 (3)	1 (50)	0 (0)
Total	72 (100%)	50 (69)	17 (24)

Abbreviations: GA, general anesthesia; MAC, monitored anesthesia care; NORA, non–operating room anesthesia.

most common drug implicated in oversedation. Propofol alone was administered in 22%, whereas propofol in combination with other medications was used in 67% of NORA claims. Reviewers judged 68% of these oversedation claims (13 cases; see **Table 5**) to be probably preventable by better monitoring. Of the 13 claims, in 12, nonuse of end-tidal CO_2 monitoring was implicated. In the remaining case, the reviewer cited poor vigilance to monitors. Substandard anesthesia care was cited in 88% of the claims (see **Table 5**). All oversedation claims (n = 20; see **Table 5**) resulted in death or permanent brain damage and payment was made to the plaintiff in 95% of claims ,with a median payment of $609,039 (see **Table 5**).

Non–Operating Room Anesthesia Care Cases in National Anesthesia Clinical Outcomes Registry Versus Claims

NORA claims constituted a significantly smaller proportion of all malpractice claims (4%) compared with the proportion of NORA cases (19%) as estimated by NACOR data (**Fig. 3**). The majority of NORA cases and claims were in the GI suite (**Fig. 4**). However, a greater portion of NORA claims occurred in radiology (19%) and cardiology (29%) compared with NACOR cases (9% and 9%, respectively; see **Fig. 4**). Patients in NORA claims were more often ASA 3 to 5 than in NACOR cases (66% in claims vs 41% NACOR cases; $P<.01$). The proportion of pediatric patients was similar in NORA claims and NACOR cases; however, the proportion of young/middle aged adults (19–49 years of age) was greater in NORA claims than in NACOR cases (31% in claims vs

Table 3
Most common complications in NORA claims versus operating room claims

	NORA Claims (N = 72), n (%)	OR Claims (N = 1828), n (%)	P Value
Death	44 (61)	556 (30)	<.001
Permanent brain damage	10 (14)	208 (11)	.308
Aspiration pneumonitis	9 (13)	80 (4)	.005
Airway injury	3 (4)	151 (8)	.150
Eye injury	2 (3)	108 (6)	.200
Pain during surgery	2 (3)	14 (1)	.121
Nerve injury	1 (1)	333 (18)	<.001
Myocardial infarction	1 (1)	75 (4)	.206

N = 1900 claims.
Abbreviations: NORA, non–operating room anesthesia; OR, operating room.

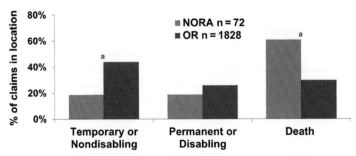

Fig. 1. Severity of injury in non–operating room anesthesia (NORA) claims compared with operating room (OR) claims. [a]P<.001.

20% in NACOR cases; $P = .02$). MAC was more often the primary anesthetic in NORA claims compared with cases (69% in claims vs 38% in NACOR cases; $P<.01$).

Preventability of Injury and Liability

A greater proportion of NORA claims than OR claims were judged to be preventable by better monitoring ($P<.001$; see **Table 1**). Anesthesia care in NORA claims was more frequently judged as substandard and NORA claims resulted in more payments and higher payments amounts ($P<.01$; see **Table 1**) than in OR claims.

DISCUSSION

We compared claims from the Anesthesia Closed Claims database with data collected from NACOR to assess for patterns of injury when comparing anesthesia care provided in remote locations compared to a traditional OR. Our data suggest a lower risk of malpractice claims in NORA compared with OR settings. Although most remote location claims and cases took place in the GI suite, radiology and cardiology locations were more frequent in malpractice claims when compared with NACOR cases. These results suggest an increased risk in radiology and cardiology NORA procedures.

Table 4
Mechanisms of injury in NORA claims versus operating room claims

	NORA Claims (N = 72), n (%)	OR Claims (N = 1828), n (%)	P Value
Respiratory events	38 (53)	416 (23)	<.001
Inadequate oxygenation/ventilation	22 (31)	116 (6)	<.001
Cardiovascular events	10 (14)	269 (15)	.505
Equipment events	7 (10)	333 (18)	.039
Regional block events	0 (0)	192 (11)	<.001
Medication-related events	4 (6)	102 (6)	.626
Other events[a]	12 (17)	485 (27)	.037

N = 1900 claims.
Abbreviations: NORA, non–operating room anesthesia; OR, operating room.
[a] Other events include surgical technique/patient condition, patient fell, wrong operation/location, positioning, failure to diagnose, other known damaging events, no damaging events, and unknown damaging events.

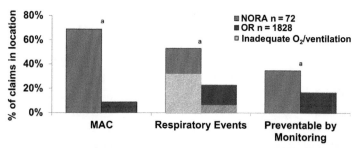

Fig. 2. Characteristics of malpractice claims in non–operating room anesthesia (NORA) locations compared with operating room (OR) locations. Hatched section of bars indicate proportion of inadequate oxygenation/ventilation as a subset of respiratory events. MAC, monitored anesthesia care; O_2, oxygenation. [a]$P<.01$.

Greater Relative Risk in Cardiology and Radiology Locations

Gastroenterology procedures in the NORA setting were less likely to be associated with a malpractice claim when compared with other NORA locations. We believe two main factors may account for this occurrence. The first is the more invasive nature

Table 5	
Characteristics of NORA claims associated with oversedation (n = 20)	
Characteristic	**n (%)**
Age > 70 y (n = 20)	3 (15)
ASA physical status 3–5 (n = 20)	14 (70)
Obese (n = 18)	12 (67)
Location (n = 20)	
Gastrointestinal suite	13 (65)
Radiology	3 (15)
Cardiology	3 (15)
Lithotripsy	1 (5)
Sedative agents (n = 18)	
Propofol plus benzodiazepines/opioids/ketamine/lidocaine	12 (67)
Propofol alone	4 (22)
Others (no propofol): benzodiazepine, opioid, ketamine	2 (11)
Preventable by better monitoring (n = 19)	
Probably	13 (68)
Would not prevent	6 (32)
Death or permanent brain damage (n = 20)	20 (100)
Substandard care (n = 17)	15 (88)
Payment to plaintiff (n = 20)	
Payment made	19 (95)
Median (interquartile range) of payments (2016$)	$609,039
25% Quartile	$298,700
75% Quartile	$1,328,700

Percentages based on claims without missing data. Denominators are listed in parentheses. Payments adjusted to 2016 dollars using the Consumer Price Index.
Abbreviations: ASA, American Society of Anesthesiologists; NORA, non–operating room anesthesia; OR, operating room.

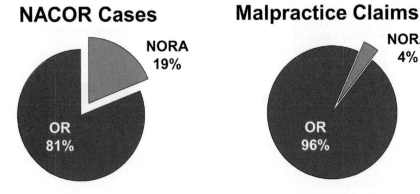

NACOR Cases

NORA
19%

OR
81%

n = 9,890,875 cases 2010–13

Malpractice Claims

NORA
4%

OR
96%

n = 1900 claims 2000–12

Fig. 3. Proportion of cases in non–operating room anesthesia (NORA) locations in the National Anesthesia Clinical Outcomes Registry (NACOR) database compared with the proportion of malpractice claims associated with NORA.

of procedures done in NORA radiology and cardiology locations. Procedures in the GI suite are usually less invasive, such as upper endoscopies and colonoscopies. The second factor is the large number of screening examinations done in the GI suite, specifically, screening colonoscopies. These cases dilute the data with a large number of healthy individuals undergoing a routine screening procedure and who are less likely to have the medical complexities of patients presenting for an intervention. Cardiology and radiology locations do not routinely require anesthesia for procedures that screen a healthy population.

Predominance of Respiratory Adverse Events and Monitoring Requirements

Adverse respiratory events were responsible for more than one-half (53%) of all closed claims filed in the NORA setting (see **Fig. 2**). Pediatrics data also showed a need for airway intervention to be fairly common in remote locations (0.5% of cases).[12]

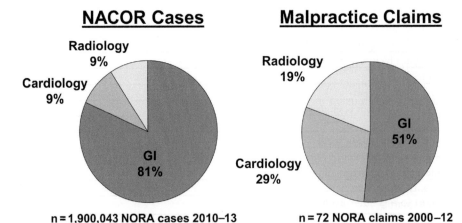

NACOR Cases

Radiology
9%

Cardiology
9%

GI
81%

n = 1,900,043 NORA cases 2010–13

Malpractice Claims

Radiology
19%

GI
51%

Cardiology
29%

n = 72 NORA claims 2000–12

Fig. 4. Location of non–operating room anesthesia (NORA) cases in the National Anesthesia Clinical Outcomes Registry (NACOR) database compared with malpractice claims. GI, gastrointestinal suite.

The greater proportion of inadequate oxygenation/ventilation in NORA claims (see **Fig. 2**) is not surprising; the majority involved MAC and the most common source of injury in MAC cases is severe respiratory depression.[13] MAC cases were significantly overrepresented in the NORA claims compared with NACOR cases (69% vs 38%; $P<.01$). However, the difference in anesthesia type may also reflect differences in classification of sedation for billing purposes in the NACOR database. A significantly greater proportion of NORA cases was judged to be preventable by better monitoring, particularly capnography which measures exhaled carbon dioxide. Improving patient monitoring in the NORA setting has become a major patient safety effort in attempts to maintain the same standards of care as those in the OR.

In the early 1990s, specialty societies and individual practitioners began to notice a significant increase in anesthesia and proceduralist-led sedation cases in nontraditional locations. Safety and quality concerns in this area lead to the 1994 statement by the ASA listing the required care elements for non–OR anesthetizing locations.[14] The ASA's goal was to bring the safety standards of the NORA environment up to those of the traditional OR. The statement was updated in 2013 and lists several requirements needed for safe anesthesia practice. These include a reliable source of oxygen, suction, a well-maintained anesthesia machine, adequate scavenging when inhalation anesthetics are administered, a hand resuscitation bag, adequate drugs and supplies, equipment to meet standards for basic monitoring, labeled outlets with an emergency power supply, proper illumination, sufficient space, immediate access to an emergency cart with a defibrillator, reliable 2-way communication, and appropriately trained staff as essential. Regardless of anesthesia or sedation depth, vital organ function monitoring is mandatory and OR standards should be met, regardless of location.[2] The ASA Standards for Basic Anesthesia Monitoring are now held as the standard for both inside and outside of the OR.[15] Organizations such as the Centers for Medicare and Medicaid Services and The Joint Commission also agree that the same standards of anesthetic administration will be observed regardless of the anesthetizing location.

Overall Safety and Risk

Challenges in maintaining NORA environment quality stem from many different sources: remote locations, increased noise during the procedure, limited work space, inadequate lighting and temperature regulation, electrical interference, older and unfamiliar equipment, and a lack of additional resources such as drugs or skilled personnel have all been implicated as challenges more common to non-OR locations.[16] Even with these challenges, our data suggest that NORA cases are less likely to involve a complication resulting in a malpractice claim (see **Fig. 3**). Our finding is consistent with the lower rate of self-reported complications in NORA compared with OR settings using the NACOR database.[9] The Pediatric Sedation Consortium data also show that when proper monitoring and trained professionals perform sedation, catastrophic events are unlikely to occur.[12]

Although overall claims seem to be lower for NORA cases, a death from a complication in a NORA setting may be more likely to result in a malpractice claim than perioperative death in the OR setting. The finding that patients aged 19 to 49 had a higher representation in claims than baseline NACOR demographic data is mostly likely related to a greater likelihood for a claim being filed on behalf of a younger patient. However, it is also possible that anesthesia providers are not being as well-prepared for complications in a younger and seemingly healthier population. Additionally, cardiac adverse events, adverse and allergic medication events, and equipment-related complications occurred in similar proportions in OR and NORA claims emphasizing that, although rare, adverse complications occur in NORA settings. The potentially serious nature of NORA complications cannot be understated and providers must be vigilant and prepared to manage emergencies at all times.

Changing Trends in Non–Operating Room Anesthesia and Opportunities for Future Data Collection

NORA is a rapidly growing area of anesthesia, but limited data exist on the demographics of NORA patients, case characteristics, outcomes, and how these are changing over time. When NORA started to gain attention in the early 1990s, sedation duties were performed by nurses and proceduralists. The NORA environment was not yet seen as a priority for anesthesia provider involvement because most of the cases were considered lower risk and less invasive. In 1994, the same year as the ASA Statement on the required elements for out of OR anesthesia was published, the faculty from the Harvard teaching hospitals published the first guidelines for sedation by non-anesthesiologists.[17] Interestingly, the guidelines noted that, although anesthesiologists have the unique qualifications to provide sedation, their primary commitments remain the intensive care unit, the pain service, and the OR environment. Since that time, NORA cases have advanced in complexity as areas such as interventional cardiology, radiology, and others have expanded into specialty non-OR procedural areas where an anesthesia provider is often needed and preferred.[9] Apart from individual hospitals' publications, until recently using the NACOR database, we have not been able to effectively track NORA case trends.[9]

Increased regulation along with the rise of value-based payment methods has led to new initiatives to improve outcome data aggregation.[18] Electronic health care records have made it much easier to collect and subsequently analyze vast amounts of information and provide analysis such as ours. Facing an evolving regulatory and reimbursement landscape, the ASA chartered the AQI in 2008 to promote quality improvement in anesthesia. A main focus of the AQI is the development of the NACOR, a major source for our data. NACOR and other emerging registries will continue to grow and collect information to be used for big data analysis. These large datasets are becoming increasingly important for linking outcomes in anesthesia to the actions that lead to them.[19] For example, a recent analysis of the NACOR database found an increase in the proportion of NORA cases compared with all anesthesia cases from 2010 to 2014, as well as delineated current trends in patient and procedure characteristics in these locations.[20]

Alternative Sources of Non–Operating Room Anesthesia Outcomes Data: Pediatric Sedation Consortium

At this time, the only other large source of NORA outcomes data comes from pediatric anesthesia. Data obtained from the Pediatric Sedation Research Consortium has given us the best information to date on the frequency and nature of complications outside of the OR. The organization's first report in 2006 included more than 35,000 pediatric sedation encounters.[12] No deaths were reported and a single instance of cardiac arrest directly associated with the anesthetic care occurred. Much more common was the need for airway intervention. One in every 200 sedations required more advanced airway management such as bag-mask ventilation or emergency intubation. More common still, 1 in 64 encounters saw oxygen saturation decrease to less than 90% for longer than 30 seconds. It was noted that the institutions included in this data collection had specialty sedation services and participated in quality improvement efforts making them likely to outperform less stringent anesthesia facilities. These pediatric results align well with our data showing that respiratory events, specifically inadequate ventilation/oxygenation, are the most common damaging events in NORA claims (see **Fig. 2**).

A subsequent report focused on sedation encounters involving propofol and remains a landmark study with detailed outcomes reported on 49,836 pediatric encounters.[21] Again, no deaths were reported but 2 cardiac arrests requiring cardiopulmonary resuscitation and 4 aspiration events were documented. One in 65 encounters involved some type of airway complication (stridor, laryngospasm, wheezing, central apnea) and 1 in 70 required a form of airway intervention. This study highlighted that complications, especially related to propofol administration, were not infrequent, but when propofol was administered in an optimized environment it rarely led to major morbidity and mortality.

Limitations in Data Comparison

Using closed claims data is inherently biased and there are some significant limitations, as described elsewhere.[7,22,23] Briefly stated, malpractice claims are a collection of infrequent, "sentinel" events that often involve substandard care and severe, permanent injuries. The data can be used to identify areas of recurrent risk and provide direction for more in-depth analysis. There is no scientifically accurate way to calculate risk, because the denominator (total number of anesthesia events) is not known. We attempted to better understand the frequency of poor outcomes by comparing the claims data to NACOR data. The NACOR data tells us the relative volume and information on anesthesia case characteristics. Using NACOR data to describe NORA trends and case volume is likely generalizable since the data included multiple settings and a broad range of patients and providers.[20] Although this does not give us an exact denominator to use with closed claims data, it does provide us with case distribution and proportions that are likely comparable.

Other obvious limitations include limiting both datasets to strict case definitions and exclusion criteria. This was done diligently, but at times remains impossible with the given information. Difference in time periods in the comparison was also a limitation. NACOR data from 2010 to 2013 were compared with closed claims data from 2000 to 2012. However, we believe the comparison is useful and a larger time period is needed for the limited number of NORA closed claims, but acknowledge changing NORA trends could be a factor.

SUMMARY

NORA continues to expand, and patient safety concerns remain given the evolution in patient and procedure complexity. Our review of closed claims and NACOR data shows that NORA malpractice claims more often involve death and substandard care when compared with the OR setting. Most NORA claims involved GI procedures; however, cardiology and radiology procedures were overrepresented in claims compared with cases in NACOR. NORA patients were more likely to be an ASA Physical Status 3 to 5 undergoing MAC, with inadequate oxygenation/ventilation responsible for nearly one-third of NORA claims. Although significant risks are associated with anesthesia in remote locations, NORA seems to be quite safe overall. Poor outcomes in closed claims reporting were often tied to suboptimal care and non-adherence to the basic safe practice principles established by the ASA. Clinicians must always be prepared for emergencies, because complications can be exceedingly difficult to manage in the NORA environments. When the quality of the environment and patient preparation are upheld, serious complications in NORA are rare.

REFERENCES

1. Ferrari LR. Anesthesia outside the operating room. Curr Opin Anaesthesiol 2015; 28:439–40.
2. Eichhorn V, Henzler D, Murphy MF. Standardizing care and monitoring for anesthesia or procedural sedation delivered outside the operating room. Curr Opin Anaesthesiol 2010;23:494–9.
3. Chang B, Urman RD. Non-operating room anesthesia: the principles of patient assessment and preparation. Anesthesiol Clin 2016;34:223–40.
4. Metzner J, Domino KB. Risks of anesthesia or sedation outside the operating room: the role of the anesthesia care provider. Curr Opin Anaesthesiol 2010;23: 523–31.
5. Robbertze R, Posner KL, Domino KB. Closed claims review of anesthesia for procedures outside the operating room. Curr Opin Anaesthesiol 2006;19:436–42.
6. Metzner J, Posner KL, Domino KB. The risk and safety of anesthesia at remote locations: the US closed claims analysis. Curr Opin Anaesthesiol 2009;22:502–8.
7. Cheney FW, Posner K, Caplan RA, et al. Standard of care and anesthesia liability. JAMA 1989;261:1599–603.
8. Cheney FW. The American Society of Anesthesiologists Closed Claims Project: what have we learned, how has it affected practice, and how will it affect practice in the future? Anesthesiology 1999;91:552–6.
9. Chang B, Kaye AD, Diaz JH, et al. Complications of non-operating room procedures: outcomes from the National Anesthesia Clinical Outcomes Registry. J Patient Saf 2015;1–7.
10. Dutton RP. Making a difference: the Anesthesia Quality Institute. Anesth Analg 2015;120:507–9.
11. Bureau of Labor Statistics US Department of Labor: Consumer Price Index inflation calculator, Bureau of Labor Statistics, US Department of Labor. Available at: http://www.bls.gov/data/home.htm. Accessed February 24, 2017.
12. Cravero JP, Blike GT, Beach M, et al. Incidence and nature of adverse events during pediatric sedation/anesthesia for procedures outside the operating room: report from the Pediatric Sedation Research Consortium. Pediatrics 2006;118: 1087–96.
13. Bhananker SM, Posner KL, Cheney FW, et al. Injury and liability associated with monitored anesthesia care: a closed claims analysis. Anesthesiology 2006;104: 228–34.
14. American Society of Anesthesiologists (ASA). ASA statement on nonoperating room anesthetizing locations. Available at: http://www.asahq.org/~/media/sites/ asahq/files/public/resources/standards-guidelines/statement-on-nonoperating-room-anesthetizing-locations.pdf. Accessed January 8, 2017.
15. American Society of Anesthesiologists (ASA). ASA standards for basic anesthetic monitoring. Available at: http://www.asahq.org/quality-and-practice-management/ standards-and-guidelines. Accessed February 26, 2017.
16. Melloni C. Anesthesia and sedation outside the operating room: how to prevent risk and maintain good quality. Curr Opin Anaesthesiol 2007;20:513–9.
17. Holzman RS, Cullen DJ, Eichhorn JH, et al. Guidelines for sedation by nonanesthesiologists during diagnostic and therapeutic procedures. The Risk Management Committee of the Department of Anaesthesia of Harvard Medical School. J Clin Anesth 1994;6:265–76.
18. Liau A, Havidich JE, Onega T, et al. The National Anesthesia Clinical Outcomes Registry. Anesth Analg 2015;121:1604–10.

19. Dutton RP. Large databases in anaesthesiology. Curr Opin Anaesthesiol 2015;28: 697–702.
20. Nagrebetsky A, Gabriel RA, Dutton RP, et al. Growth of nonoperating room anesthesia care in the United States: a contemporary trends analysis. Anesth Analg 2017;124:1261–7.
21. Cravero JP, Beach ML, Blike GT, et al, Pediatric Sedation Research Consortium. The incidence and nature of adverse events during pediatric sedation/anesthesia with propofol for procedures outside the operating room: a report from the Pediatric Sedation Research Consortium. Anesth Analg 2009;108:795–804.
22. Caplan RA, Posner KL, Cheney FW. Effect of outcome on physician judgments of appropriateness of care. JAMA 1991;265:1957–60.
23. Lee LA, Domino KB. The Closed Claims Project. Has it influenced anesthetic practice and outcome? Anesthesiol Clin North America 2002;20:485–501.

Implementation and Use of Anesthesia Information Management Systems for Non–operating Room Locations

Jason T. Bouhenguel, MD, MS[a], David A. Preiss, MD, PhD[a],
Richard D. Urman, MD, MBA, FASA[a,b,*]

KEYWORDS

- Electronic health record • Implementation
- Anesthesia information management system • Non-operating room • Anesthesia
- Electronic medical record • EPIC

KEY POINTS

- Demand for anesthesia services in non–operating room sites increases as procedures of increasing complexity are being offered to patients of increasing comorbidity.
- Despite financial and logistical obstacles to implementation of anesthesia information management systems and electronic medical records, the benefits to non–operating room anesthesia services outweigh the costs.
- Access to a patient's electronic medical record facilitates preoperative evaluation, allowing for advanced review of patient medical history, labs, medications, and studies.
- Intraoperative assistance promotes a smoother intraoperative anesthesia workflow while potentially improving the quality of anesthesia care delivered and overall patient safety.

INTRODUCTION

The ongoing widespread adoption of anesthesia information management systems (AIMS) has been in large part due to the incentives and mandates set forth by the Health Information Technology for Economic and Clinical Health Act and the Electronic Health Record (EHR) Incentive Program of 2009. Despite our initial motivation for adoption, however, the usefulness of these AIMS solutions is becoming far greater

Disclosures: None.
[a] Department of Anesthesiology, Perioperative and Pain Medicine, Brigham and Women's Hospital, 75 Francis Street, Boston, MA 02115, USA; [b] Center for Perioperative Research, Brigham and Women's Hospital, 75 Francis Street, Boston, MA 02115, USA
* Corresponding author. Department of Anesthesiology, Perioperative and Pain Medicine, Brigham and Women's Hospital, 75 Francis Street, Boston, MA 02115.
E-mail address: rurman@bwh.harvard.edu

Anesthesiology Clin 35 (2017) 583–590
http://dx.doi.org/10.1016/j.anclin.2017.07.001
1932-2275/17/© 2017 Elsevier Inc. All rights reserved.

than previously anticipated, especially in the coordination and delivery of anesthesia care outside of the operating room (OR).

Non–operating room anesthesia (NORA) accounts for nearly 40% of all anesthesiologists' workload.[1] Composed of a heterogeneous mixture of interventional and diagnostic as well as urgent and elective encounters, NORA stretches beyond the framework of conventional ORs and into interventional and endoscopic suites, outpatient offices, and obstetrics labor and delivery wards, as well as radiographic imaging centers (**Box 1**).

With the advent of newer, less-invasive procedures, proceduralists are able to offer medically challenging patients increasingly more complex interventions outside of the OR. Patients exhibiting chronic comorbid conditions including obstructive sleep apnea, obesity, heart disease (eg, coronary artery disease, congestive heart failure, arrhythmias, structural heart disease), or chronic pulmonary disease pose significant periprocedural risks, raising concerns of patient safety in these locations that may have limited staffing or necessary resuscitation or monitoring equipment. The presence of anesthesia providers can facilitate procedure throughput and help to optimize medical conditions in this patient population.[2]

The increased presence of anesthesia providers outside of the conventional OR setting, however, has placed strains on both anesthesiologists as well as the care delivery system. Complicated preprocedural evaluations, less-than-ideal physical workspaces, lack of an AIMS system, and limited on-site resources including technical support are only a few of the issues that may be encountered by NORA providers.[3]

Despite the initial obstacles inherent to implementation and maintenance of current AIMS and EHR solutions (**Box 2**),[4] numerous benefits have materialized, allowing for

---

Box 1
Examples of non–operating room anesthetizing sites

Radiology
- Interventional
- MRI
- Computer tomography
- Ultrasound
- Radiation oncology

Gastroenterology

Cardiac interventions
- Electrophysiology
- Catheterization
- Interventional cardiology
- Transesophageal echocardiography

Lithotripsy

Electroconvulsive therapy sites

Emergency room

Intensive care units

Obstetric labor and delivery

Hospital wards

Ambulatory procedure rooms

Outpatient offices

Box 2
Obstacles to implementation of AIMS/EHR solutions

1. Large capital investment.

2. Steep learning curves inherent to adoption of new technologies.

3. Maintenance, system updates, and system downtime.

4. No "one-size-fits-all" solution.
    Site-specific workflows and documentation requirements makes implementation and adoption more nuanced and complicated.

5. Integration and cross-talk of third-party systems.
    Equipment is not standardized; AIMS/EHRs must be capable of interfacing with a variety of third-party applications and devices to facilitate integration into preexisting environments.

Abbreviations: AIMS, anesthesia information management system; EHR, electronic health record.

---

more efficient, safe, and effective delivery of NORA.[5] From more efficient and comprehensive preprocedure coordination and intraprocedure aids, to streamlined postprocedure documentation and billing mechanics, AIMS solutions continue to add to our ever-expanding toolkit.

PREOPERATIVE WORKFLOW
Replacing the Paper Chart

Given the ambulatory nature and perceived "minimal-ness" of many out-of-OR procedures, scheduled patients frequently undergo little to no "anesthesia or preoperative" evaluation before the day of the procedure. In fact, these patients are often referred from outside physicians and are not only new to the anesthesia provider, but to the proceduralist as well. In a time not too long ago (and in some hospitals and procedure centers not too far away), an anesthesiologist's preoperative ritual consisted of thumbing through a patient's paper chart, teasing out as much relevant medical history as possible in the few minutes just before the start of a case. Since the advent and implementation of AIMS and EHRs, much, if not all of a patient's medical and surgical history is made available electronically in a searchable, predictable format, allowing for preprocedural evaluations to be performed by the anesthesiologist in an time-efficient manner, often before even meeting the patient.[6]

Quick and reliable access to a patient's history allows for easy review of prior anesthetic events, pertinent acute or chronic medical conditions, recent laboratory values and other studies, and active medications. Rather than thumbing through a medical maze, we are able to glean a more comprehensive medical history in a timely manner, making it less likely that we miss important facts.

Increasing Preparedness and Reducing Delays

Preprocedure knowledge of anesthesia-specific information, such as a previously difficult airway, intraoperative hemodynamic instability (eg cardiac arrhythmia, hypotension), bronchospasm, or a history of malignant hyperthermia, for example, would allow us to be better prepared for subsequent encounters. Other valuable patient-specific information readily available in the patient's AIMS and EHR record may include unfulfilled orders, active medications, code status, or the identity of a patient's health care proxy. Having this information at our fingertips can help us to identify and quickly address issues such as missing preprocedure laboratories, inappropriately continued or held medications, and incomplete anesthesia or procedural consent before the intended procedure. Our ability to perform preliminary review of patient information in this way has not only led to improved safety and preoperative preparedness, but also reduced delays and/or cancelations for reasons of inappropriate laboratory values, missing information, or the need for further medical assessment.[7–9]

Facilitating Emergent Procedures

This ease of access to a patient's comprehensive medical record becomes vitally important in the setting of emergent or impromptu procedures in which anesthesiologists and interventionists alike have little to no time to acquire outside medical records or communicate with patients regarding their active medical issues. Access to the latest laboratory values, recent echocardiography reports and electrocardiograms, and a current medication list can serve as life-saving information in times of emergency.[10]

INTRAPROCEDURE WORKFLOW

NORA facilities present various layouts, such as the placement of imaging equipment, anesthesia machine and monitors, sometimes hindering access to the patient or equipment, potentially compromising patient safety. Although general anesthesia could be considered as the "great enabler of modern day surgery," because it developed along with surgical advancement in the OR (both figuratively and literally), this is not the case for many non-OR procedures. The recent incorporation of general anesthesia or "monitored anesthesia care" into these practice settings often feels like an afterthought.

Challenging Work Environments

First, many of the NORA facilities were not designed for their current use, let alone the addition of anesthesia support. Even those spaces that were intentionally designed to complement their intervention (such as interventional cardiology or neuroradiology suites) tend to be so interventionalist-centric that the addition of anesthesia equipment and anesthesia providers can be described as inconvenient at best. Often, anesthesia equipment is relegated to tight corners and the anesthesia provider has limited to no access to the patient. These cramped, less-than-ideal workspaces contribute to a variety of inefficiencies and disruptions in the anesthetic workflow, leading to difficulties in multitasking between intraoperative documentation, patient care, and crisis management.

NORA facilities, by their very nature are frequently removed from the ORs and the typical OR support staff. Greater physical distances from fellow anesthesia care providers, anesthesia technicians, pharmacists, and surgical colleagues introduce barriers to timely support and thus increased risk of delay in case of an emergency.[11] More than usual, preparedness and communication in these settings is of the utmost importance.

AIMS and EHR solutions facilitate delivery of anesthesia outside of the OR by offloading simple but resource-intensive tasks such as intraprocedure documentation and care coordination between providers and support staff, as well by providing intraprocedure reminders and decision support tools.

Intraprocedure Documentation

Intraprocedure data collection and documentation is a major responsibility of the anesthesia provider. A key feature of many high-end AIMS solutions (eg EPIC, Cerner,

MediTech) is automated data collection. Capable of being configured to interface with numerous peripheral devices either locally or over the facility network, AIMS is able to automatically fetch and record a variety of intraprocedure information from patient-specific vitals, to ventilator settings and anesthetic measurements. A responsibility that once lay solely on the shoulders of the anesthesia provider can now be outsourced to a computer, allowing the providers to focus their attention more completely on patient care rather than the accuracy of their medical chart.[12]

Automated intraoperative documentation and easy-to-use procedure templates (eg, peripheral nerve blocks, neuraxial techniques, line placement) further facilitate timely completion of essential documents necessary for provider compliance measures and patient billing.

Support Aids

Some AIMS solutions also incorporate intraprocedure features such as triggered cascades, reminders, and decision support tools to assist the anesthesia provider in providing systematic and conscientious patient-specific care. Reminders regarding patient allergies, drug–drug interactions, and patient-specific contraindications to medication administration to help ensure patient safety. Particularly when paired with medication management systems, such as the BD Intelliport (Becton Dickinson, Franklin Lakes, NJ), it becomes theoretically possible to completely eliminate medication administration errors. Triggered cascades, or event-triggered macros, are additional tools AIMS solutions offer to assist providers in complying with tasks such as antibiotic redosing and timely intraprocedure administration of other medications.

Further intraprocedure decision support and crisis detection aids are being developed to assist in early recognition and detection of high morbidity and mortality events such as adverse cardiopulmonary events (eg myocardial infarction, pulmonary embolism, pneumothorax, bronchospasm) or adverse medication reactions (eg malignant hyperthermia or anaphylaxis), and to help guide the anesthetic regimen in real time.[13]

Care Coordination

AIMS and EHRs are being used to help coordinate care among health care providers, including pharmacists and nurses, in addition to ancillary support staff such as laboratories and blood banks. Features such as integration of third-party paging systems, in which AIMS and EHRs are capable of sending pages to support staff on behalf of active users helps to minimize time lost in time-sensitive situations. Remote access to real-time intraoperative records via networked computers or mobile devices further streamlines communication between the staff directly providing patient care and support staff behind the scenes. The ability for attending physicians or supervising anesthesia staff to assess patient stability and appropriateness of care (such as the administration of medications or blood products) remotely while supervising anesthetic care for multiple rooms or on-going procedures ensures closer supervision and the ability to offer support quickly without prompting.

CURRENT ISSUES AND FUTURE DIRECTIONS

Although AIMS solutions have added a number of tools to our anesthesia toolkit facilitating the NORA experience, there remain a variety of issues to be addressed and further advances to be made.

Anesthesia Information Management Systems

Implementation of AIMS comprises multiple phases, typically divided into preimplementation, implementation, and postimplementation, spanning the course of multiple months.[14] During the preimplementation phase, pertinent physical components (eg, anesthesia machines, ventilators, and patient data modules [PDMs] and patient vital monitors) are identified and software drivers are secured. Communication between the new AIMS and the new or preexisting EHR is established, and the new pairing is tested and validated in a sandbox test environment, ensuring a high fidelity of documentation and system stability under standard use conditions. The go-live of the AIMS is best achieved with a staged roll out—ensuring workstations are updated, connected, and consistent across the entire platform. During the postimplementation phase, issues involving system failures and ongoing user feedback is addressed while routine maintenance and system upgrades are implemented, ensuring the highest level of system stability possible.

There are several reasons why a clinician could encounter difficulties when working with a newly installed AIMS. First, the system may have bugs or errors that prevent the user from documenting properly or safely. Second, the user may not possess adequate training to confidently use it.

One of the ways one may measure the quality of EHR adoption is to determine the number of cases in which documentation reverts to a backup system, which was a paper record in the case of our hospital. At our institution, we examined the number of times a paper record was documented in our hospital across 4 areas: obstetrics, interventional procedural areas (radiology, gastroenterology, cardiology), inpatient floor and intensive care units, and the main OR. Because initial implementation is usually associated with the most problems, we examined the first 4 weeks after go-live, as well as 1-month periods from that point on. From these results, it seems that the first month required the most conversions to paper records in all areas. In the first month, anesthesia cases in the interventional procedural areas required conversion to paper 93 times, a far greater number than any other area (**Table 1**). By the second month, paper records were being used very infrequently.

Table 1
Incidence of reversion to paper charting, as a function of time from day of go-live of the institutional AIMS

	Obstetrics	Interventional Procedural Areas	Inpatient Floor/ICU	Main OR
Days from go-live				
7	3	22	0	0
14	0	20	1	0
21	0	29	0	1
28	0	22	0	0
Months from go-live				
1	3	93	1	1
2	1	3	0	1
3	1	3	1	0
4	0	3	0	0

Abbreviations: AIMS, anesthesia information management system; ICU, intensive care unit; OR, operating room.

Although we present only absolute numbers and not percentages, these data suggest that EHR implementation in the interventional procedural areas posed greater problems to our clinicians than in the main OR. These problems were largely corrected by the second month.

The reason for this difference could be either inadequate staff education or technical malfunctions with equipment unique to the interventional procedural areas. Our anesthesia team frequently alternates their staffing location such that the same team floats from the main OR to non-OR locations, so the hypothesis that individual training was inadequate should not apply. It is therefore more likely that the EHR created more technical challenges in the non-OR environment than in the main OR. This may be due to either hardware incompatibility with the new EHR, or a less intuitive workflow for the clinicians.

Steep Learning Curves

AIMS and EHRs in their current forms are often cumbersome products with steep learning curves. Navigating the wealth of information contained within an AIMS and EHR system is no easy feat. Numerous tabs within a patient chart, a variety of different appearing provider-specific workspaces, and countless ways of viewing the same patient information tend to serve as obstacles rather than features of current state-of-the-art AIMS and EHRs. Development of more ergonomic solutions and allowing for intuitive navigation of a patient's chart will further facilitate our ability to care for patients more efficiently.

Siloed Services

For starters, current AIMS and EHR platforms are fairly siloed from one another. First, there are brand barriers—EPIC versus Cerner versus MediTech—through which transfer of patient information proves to be impossible. Second, there are extrainstitutional barriers as well, where out-of-partnership electronic records still need to be transferred manually via email, fax, or a scanned physical document rather than being accessed electronically. These types of barriers need to be broken down to facilitate more efficient, less redundant, and safer delivery of care.[5] A major effort of the government mandate (Health Information Technology for Economic and Clinical Health Act) is to create a central shared repository of patient information, to be available for access across the country.

Plug and Play

Wireless vital monitors will soon replace current wired solutions and help declutter an already cramped workspace. As device integration is improved and standardized, more third-party devices will be made available with easy pairing strategies, making adoption of new technologies and monitoring systems within NORA settings easier.

Real-Time Decision Aids

Further development of real-time decision aids and crisis prediction algorithms based on automatically imported patient vitals, anesthesia machine measurements, and laboratory values will provide additional intraoperative support in caring for individual patients, particularly in less than ideal practice environments.

SUMMARY

NORA encounters comprise an impressive fraction of contemporary anesthesia practice. Many out of the OR environments suffer from a variety of limitations and constraints, hindering our ability to provide the highest and safest level of anesthesia care. Despite the large personal and financial commitments involved in adoption and implementation of AIMS and EHRs in these settings, the benefits to safety, efficacy, and efficiency are far too great to be ignored. We can better streamline the preoperative assessment via remotely available medical records, maximizing patient safety while minimizing revenue lost—owing to day-of-procedure delays and cancellations. Intraoperative assistance in the form of automated documentation, real-time decision aids, and remote real-time surveillance facilitates intraoperative workflow while potentially improving the quality of anesthesia care delivered and overall patient safety. Continued future innovation of the AIMS experience only promises to further improve on our NORA experience.

REFERENCES

1. Schubert A, Eckhout GV, Ngo AL, et al. Status of the anesthesia workforce in 2011: evolution during the last decade and future outlook. Anesth Analg 2012; 115:407–27.
2. Nagrebetsky A, Gabriel RA, Dutton RP, et al. Growth of nonoperating room anesthesia care in the United States: a contemporary trends analysis. Anesth Analg 2017;124(4):1261–7.
3. Kiekkas P. Anesthesia outside the operating room in adults: a matter of safety? Guest editorial. J Perianesth Nurs 2015;30:82–4.
4. Brovman E, Preiss D, Urman R. The challenges of implementing electronic health records for anesthesia use outside the operating room. Curr Opin Anaesthesiol 2006;29(4):531–5.
5. Gottlieb O. Anesthesia information management systems in the ambulatory setting: benefits and challenges. Anesthesiol Clin 2014;32:559–76.
6. Klafta JM, Roizen MF. Current understanding of patients' attitudes toward and preparation for anesthesia: a review. Anesth Analg 1996;83:1314–21.
7. Wu A, Kodali BS, Flanagan HL Jr, et al. Introduction of a new electronic medical record system has mixed effects on first surgical case efficiency metrics. J Clin Monit Comput 2016. [Epub ahead of print].
8. Holt NF, Silverman DG, Prasad R, et al. Preanesthesia clinics, information management, and operating room delays: results of a survey of practicing anesthesiologists. Anesth Analg 2007;104:615–8.
9. McDowell J, Wu A, Ehrenfeld JM, et al. Effect of the implementation of a new electronic health record system on surgical case turnover time. J Med Syst 2017; 41(3):42.
10. Chang B, Urman R. NORA: the principles of patient assessment and preparation. Anesthesiol Clin 2016;43(1):223–40.
11. Chang B, Kaye AD, Diaz JH, et al. Complications of non-operating room & procedures: outcomes from the National Anesthesia Clinical Outcomes Registry. J Patient Saf 2015. [Epub ahead of print].
12. Edsall DW, Deshane P, Giles C, et al. Computerized patient anesthesia records: less time and better quality than manually produced anesthesia records. J Clin Anesth 1993;4:275–83.
13. Balust J, Macario A. Can anesthesia information management systems improve quality in the surgical suite? Curr Opin Anaesthesiol 2009;22:215–22.
14. Mudumbai SC. Implementation of an anesthesia information management system in an ambulatory surgery center. J Med Syst 2016;40:22.

Monitoring for Nonoperating Room Anesthesia

Stylianos Voulgarelis, MD[a,b], John P. Scott, MD[c,d,*]

KEYWORDS

- Monitoring • Nonoperating room anesthesia • Office-based anesthesia
- Capnography

KEY POINTS

- Regardless of the depth of anesthesia provided, it is of paramount importance that all providers administering anesthesia at a remote location adhere to the American Society of Anesthesiologists (ASA) guidelines for standard monitoring.
- The ASA recommends the assessment of oxygenation, ventilation, and circulation during any anesthetic regardless the location or type of anesthetic.
- The use of invasive or noninvasive advanced monitors depends on the complexity of the procedure or the patient's history.

INTRODUCTION

Procedures requiring nonoperating room anesthesia (NORA) have increased in quantity and complexity during the last 20 years.[1] The etiology of this phenomenon is multifactorial, related to technological advancements, health care improvement, and evolving expectations of patients and providers. Technological advancements have driven new diagnostic, therapeutic, and palliative interventions in order to improve quality of life. Life expectancy has increased, resulting in older more complex patients requiring procedures previously reserved for healthy patients who may not have required sedation. Anesthetic delivery is generally regarded as safe due to technological and pharmacologic improvements, and many nonanesthesiologists now routinely

Disclosure Statement: None.
[a] Division of Pediatric Anesthesiology, Medical College of Wisconsin, Milwaukee, WI, USA;
[b] Division of Adult Cardiac Anesthesiology, Medical College of Wisconsin, Milwaukee, WI, USA; [c] Anesthesiology, Division of Pediatric Anesthesiology, Pediatric Intensive Care Unit, Children's Hospital of Wisconsin, MCW, Milwaukee, WI, USA; [d] Pediatrics, Division of Pediatric Critical Care, Pediatric Intensive Care Unit, Children's Hospital of Wisconsin, MCW, Milwaukee, WI, USA
* Corresponding author. 9000 West Wisconsin Avenue, PO Box 1997, MS 735, Milwaukee, WI 53201-3022.
E-mail address: scottjake@mcw.edu

Anesthesiology Clin 35 (2017) 591–599
http://dx.doi.org/10.1016/j.anclin.2017.07.004
anesthesiology.theclinics.com

provide sedation.[2] Consequently, personnel working in these locations may not have the advanced training necessary to care for complex patients in nonoperating room settings. The roles of anesthesiologists as members of care teams in nonoperating room locations continue to evolve. Anesthesia providers are now recognized as essential members of health care teams in areas where functions and responsibilities of anesthesia providers had not been previously established or recognized.

The logistics of care delivery in remote locations are complex, as each environment has is unique characteristics and safety requirements (MRI, radiotherapy, gamma-knife). Small procedure suites may not have been originally designed to accommodate anesthesia equipment or providers. New construction of remote locations must have space to accommodate for anesthesia equipment and providers. The safety of anesthetic delivery in remote locations has been enhanced through development of area-specific equipment including nonferromagnetic MRI equipment. The introduction of the electronic health record has improved provider access to patient records, augmenting preoperative assessments while also increasing the efficiency of procedural data collection. Finally, communication between remote locations and the central operating room has been enhanced, with cellular phones and vocera devices for use in emergencies or situations when additional experienced providers are needed.

Closed claims analyses have consistently identified respiratory events as the most common adverse events during NORA, occurring twice as commonly as in the operating room.[3,4] Care was described as suboptimal in 54% of the cases and the event preventable in 32% of cases. Monitored care anesthesia (MAC) was the anesthetic technique in half of the cases. Inadequate oxygenation and ventilation were the most common sources of adverse events.[5] Risk factors associated with complications were extreme of age, ASA-PS of at least 3, obesity, and emergency procedures. Remote location events were associated with more severe injuries (death and neurologic injury).

The American Society of Anesthesiologists (ASA) categorizes sedation in 4 categories, including minimal, moderate and deep sedation and general anesthesia. Only physician anesthesiologists, certified nurse anesthetists (CRNAs) and anesthesia assistants (AAs) are permitted to provide general anesthesia. Sedation may be provided by a heterogeneous group of providers with different training, skills, knowledge and practice patterns, including but not limited to other physicians, dentists, and podiatrists. Regardless of the depth of anesthesia provided, it is of paramount importance that all providers administering anesthesia at a remote location adhere to the ASA guidelines for standard monitoring. The ASA recommends the assessment of oxygenation, ventilation, and circulation during any anesthetic regardless of the location or type of anesthetic. This includes the use of continuous pulse oximetry, capnography, electrocardiogram (ECG), intermittent noninvasive blood pressure, and temperature. The use of invasive or noninvasive advanced monitors depends on the complexity of the procedure or the patient's history.

PULSE OXIMETRY

The introduction of continuous pulse oximetry in the1980s reduced the incidence of unrecognized periprocedural hypoxemia. Continuous pulse oximetry remains an essential monitor and is required by the ASA for all categories of sedation. The principals of pulse oximetry are based the Beer-Lambert law and the variable absorption of wavelengths of light by different species of hemoglobin (oxyhemoglobin (Hbo_2), deoxyhemoglobin (HbR), methemoglobin (metHb) and carboxyhemoglobin (COHb)).[6] Hbo_2 absorbs near infrared light at a wavelength of 940 nm, and HbR absorbs red light at a wavelength of 660 nm.[6] The arterial saturation is calculated as the relative ratio of red and infrared light absorption.[7]

Pulse oximetry measurement relies on pulsatile blood flow rendering it less reliable during physiologic states of reduced pulsatility such low cardiac output or extreme vasoconstriction. Absence of pulsatile blood flow during cardiopulmonary bypass or with mechanical assist devices (extracorporeal membrane oxygenation [ECMO], ventricular assist devices [VADs]) may also reduce pulse oximeter signal.[8] Interference with the transmission or absorption of light wavelengths emitted by the pulse oximeter may also produce erroneous readings. Sources of interference include nail polish or dyes used perioperatively (methylene blue, indigo carmine). Abnormal hemoglobin variants may also be associated with abnormal pulse oximeter readings.

CAPNOGRAPHY

Capnography is the continuous measurement of the partial pressure of carbon dioxide (CO_2) during inspiration and expiration. The principals of capnography rely on absorption of infrared radiation by the molecules of CO_2. The amount of infrared radiation absorbed is exponentially related to the partial pressure of CO_2.[9] The measured partial pressure of CO_2 at the end of exhalation is defined as the end tidal CO_2 ($ETCO_2$).

Prior to capnography, the assessment of ventilation relied on visual inspection and impedance plethysmography, which are insensitive for identification of hypoventilation. Room air pulse oximetry may provide some assessment of the adequacy of ventilation, but supplemental oxygen blunts detection of hypoventilation by increasing alveolar oxygen content. Capnography provides quantitative and qualitative information regarding the adequacy of ventilation.[9] Studies of adult and pediatric patients undergoing NORA have shown that capnography detects hypopnea earlier that pulse oximeter and decreases the incidence of hypoxemia.[10-14]

Capnography provides quantitative and qualitative data.[9] Hypoventilation during sedation exhibits 2 patterns. Bradypneic hypoventilation, common with opioid administration, is easily detected by capnographic tracings, demonstrating decreased rate and increased $ETCO_2$. Hypopneic hypoventilation secondary to hypnotic administration (ie, propofol) is characterized by both decreased tidal volume and respiratory rate. A significant proportion of each exhaled breath is dead space ventilation resulting in a widened arterial CO_2 to $ETCO_2$ gradient.[9]

Capnography in MAC anesthetics during NORA enables the detection of hypoventilation before it is detected by pulse oximetry. In pediatric studies of sedation in the emergency room and in MRI, capnography detected hypopneic hypoventilation 2 to 3 minutes before pulse oximetry.[10,11] Similarly in adults, capnography has been shown to provide early detection of hypoventilation and decrease the incidence of hypoxemia.[13,14]

Capnographic waveform morphology in intubated patients provides information about upper or lower airway obstruction, rebreathing of exhaled CO_2, and leak of the circuit. The $ETCO_2$ gives valuable information about circulation, perfusion, and metabolism. Hypermetabolic states (malignant hyperthermia, thyrotoxicosis, pheochromocytoma, and sepsis) may also be identified by an increase in $ETCO_2$. Additionally, decreased exhaled CO_2 may occur with pulmonary hypoperfusion caused by profound shock, low cardiac output, pulmonary embolism, or venous air embolism.[15]

ELECTROCARDIOGRAM

ECG provides the graphic representation of cardiac electrical activity including rate and rhythm. ECG monitoring is critical for early detection and diagnosis of myocardial ischemia, dysrhythmias, or critical electrolyte disturbances such as hyperkalemia or hypocalcemia.[15] The ECG does not monitor cardiac output, contractility, or oxygen delivery. Five-lead (4 leads plus fifth precordial [V5]) ECG monitoring is recommended for adult patients. The most common leads monitored are the II and V5. Lead II is useful to assess atrial conduction and detect arrhythmias and inferior wall ischemia, while lead V helps identify anterior and lateral wall ischemia.[15]

NONINVASIVE BLOOD PRESSURE

Noninvasive blood pressure measurements should be performed at least every 5 minutes during anesthesia care regardless of procedural location. The appropriate size blood pressure cuff should be chosen and most frequently is placed around the upper arm. The principles of NIBP monitoring are based on oscillometry. During cuff inflation, complete arterial compression occurs, preventing antegrade blood flow, at which point the cuff is gradually deflated. As blood flow resumes in the partially compressed artery, oscillations develop. The point of maximal oscillations defines the MAP. The systolic blood pressure (SBP) and diastolic blood pressure (DBP) are calculated based on specific algorithms. Noninvasive blood pressure (NIBP) measurement is less accurate than invasive arterial blood pressure monitoring and has been shown to overestimate blood pressure during hypotension and underestimate blood pressure during hypertension.[16]

TEMPERATURE

According to the ASA, temperature monitoring is indicated "when clinically significant changes in body temperature are intended, anticipated or suspected." The axilla, nasopharynx, esophagus, rectum, and bladder are all acceptable sites for temperature measurement.[17] Although hyperthermia may be a harbinger of malignant hyperthermia, the most common temperature abnormality is hypothermia. Most anesthetics induce a state of poikilothermia. Hypothermia is prevalent in remote locations that lack patient heating systems or require ambient cooling to prevent equipment overheating.[18] The most common mode of heat loss during anesthesia is radiant heat loss. Perioperative hypothermia has been linked to multisystem morbidity including myocardial ischemia, surgical site infections, coagulation disorders, prolonged length of hospital stay, and increased overall cost.[17–21] Methods utilized to maintain normothermia and minimize cold stress should be available in remote location, such as warmed rooms, heat lamps, intravenous fluid warmers, and heated forced air blankets.

ADVANCED MONITORS
Invasive Intravascular Monitoring

Invasive intravascular monitoring systems require percutaneous catheter placement (arterial, central venous, or pulmonary artery) and a transducer. These monitors enable the continuous beat-to-beat assessment of arterial or venous pressures.[15] Intra-arterial blood pressure monitoring is indicated for complex endovascular procedures in interventional radiology (endovascular aneurism repair [EVAR], thoracic endovascular aortic repair [TEVAR], cerebral aneurysm coil placement) and the cardiac catheterization laboratory. Arterial pressure waveforms provide information about intravascular volume, strength of the cardiac systole, compliance of the arterial bed, and competency of the aortic valve. Central venous pressure monitoring may be used to assess right ventricular end diastolic pressure (RVEDP), pulmonary capillary wedge pressure (PCWP), and left ventricular end diastolic pressure (LVEDP) if no valvular problems exist, and the pulmonary vascular resistance in normal. Central venous pressure (CVP) is not a reliable measure of intravascular volume status and should not be used in isolation to guide fluid resuscitation.[22] Central venous access is also necessary to administer potent vasoactive or inotropic medications. Large bore introducers should be placed when massive blood loss or need for transvenous pacing is anticipated. Pulmonary artery catheters (PACs) may be used for selected cardiac cases and adult liver transplants. In the remote anesthesia environment, PAC should only be used by experienced providers taking care of patients with left or right ventricular failure or liver transplant physiology.

Near Infrared Spectroscopy

Near infrared spectroscopy (NIRS) is a noninvasive method used to assess regional tissue oxygen delivery and organ perfusion. NIRS probes contain a near infrared light source and 2 receivers, calculating the regional oxygen saturation (RSO_2) based on absorption of near infrared light by hemoglobin species. The RSO_2 is a mean tissue oxyhemoglobin saturation, which may be used as a surrogate for regional venous saturation.[23] This RSO_2 value provides information regarding the regional oxygen delivery and consumption and can identify organ hypoperfusion before other manifestations of end organ dysfunction.[24]

The major limitation of NIRS monitoring is depth of near infrared light tissue penetration, which is 2 to 6 cm depending on the size of probe. Consequently, NIRS monitoring in adult patients is typically restricted to the cerebral circulation in order to assess cerebral perfusion and blood flow. For adult NORA procedures, bilateral cerebral RSO_2 monitoring has been used in interventional neuroradiology to detect critical changes in cerebral blood flow and oxygen delivery during endovascular procedures.[25] In contrast to adults, 2-site cerebral and somatic NIRS monitoring has been used in children to measure tissue saturations in the brain, kidney, and mesentery. For children with congenital heart disease, 2-site NIRS has become a widely accepted standard monitor of regional perfusion both in the operating room and ICU following open-heart surgery and cardiac catheterization procedures. Similarly NIRS can be used in the care of critically ill children who undergo remote procedures, in order to monitor the oxygen delivery. It is also important to note that bilirubin absorbs the near infrared light, making the device inaccurate in patients with jaundice.

Bispectral Index Monitoring

Bispectral index (BIS) monitoring was developed to assess depth of anesthesia and reduce awareness during surgery. The BIS index, measured 0 to 100, incorporates continuous electroencephalographic (EEG) and electromyographic (EMG) data and corresponds to the patient's level of consciousness, with values of 0 correlating to isoelectricity and 100 correlating normal awake state brain activity.[26] BIS values less than 60 are predictive general anesthesia and reduced awareness.[27] BIS monitoring may be useful in the titration of hypnotic medications in NORA, especially in vulnerable patients. Cochrane database reviews of BIS monitoring suggest that BIS monitoring has been linked to reduced anesthetic requirement, patient recall, time to extubation, and recovery time.[27]

SITE-SPECIFIC MONITORING CONSIDERATIONS
Magnetic Resonance Imaging

MRI is sensitive to motion artifact and requires varying degrees of anesthesia for patients who cannot lie still because of pain (eg, herniated disk) or anxiety. Almost all conventional monitoring devices contain ferromagnetic material and are not MRI compatible. Equipment with ferromagnetic materials pose a burn risk at areas of contact with patient. Standard ECG monitoring is not reliable because of electromagnetic distortion. ECG devices currently used subtract the electromagnetic interference, but may not be used for ST segment analysis or the detection of myocardial ischemia. Other ASA monitors are largely unaffected, but fiberoptic cables or wireless devices are required.[28] Transducers for invasive pressure monitoring contain copper, which is MRI compatible, but they should be kept off the MRI bed to reduce artifact and limit interference.[29] Hypothermia is common during MRI scanning, and temperature monitoring is indicated in children and during general anesthetics; the temperature set point within the MRI suite may not be adjusted, as this will lead to magnet malfunction.[18]

Endoscopy Suite

The ASA closed claims' analysis for remote locations identified an increased complication rate for endoscopy suite procedures. Patients older than 70 years with an ASA-PS of at least 3 are at highest risk. Most events were respiratory and mostly associated with lack of capnographic monitoring. Diminished airway reflexes with topical anesthesia and intravenous sedation increase aspiration risk, and airway obstruction may occur with placement on the endoscope. Prone positioning common during ERCP also limits access to the patient's airway. The implementation of capnography in the endoscopic suite has reduced adverse events and cost of care, significantly improving patient safety.[30] Hemodynamic lability secondary to hypovolemia should also be expected for patients who have had a bowel preparation or have active gastrointestinal bleeding.[31]

Cardiac Catheterization Laboratory

Historically, procedures performed in the cardiac catheterization of adults were limited to percutaneous coronary interventions (PCIs) for coronary artery disease and electrophysiology (EP) studies for dysrhythmias. Over last decade, the evolution in percutaneous transcatheter aortic valve replacement (TAVR) and mitral valve clipping has given the opportunity to patients who are poor surgical candidates to undergo procedures that can improve their quality of life and prolong their survival. These patients remain at high risk for perioperative morbidity and mortality. The choice of the monitors is dictated by the nature of the procedure and the physical status of the patient. For valve replacement or repair procedures, arterial and central access, as well as transesophageal echocardiogram, are recommended.

Children with complex congenital heart disease commonly require multiple cardiac catheterization procedures. Depending on ASA-PS and procedural complexity, advanced invasive as well as noninvasive monitoring may be required. NIRS monitoring provides a reliable measurement of oxygen delivery and consumption for children with heart disease.[32] Specifically, 2-site cerebral and somatic regional may be used to assess organ-specific oxygen delivery and cardiac output to vascular regions under differing mechanisms of vascular tone.[24]

Hyperbaric Oxygen Chamber

Hyperbaric oxygen (HbO) therapy may be utilized for nonhealing ulcers in diabetic patients, carbon monoxide poisoning, necrotizing soft tissue infections, and air embolus. There are 2 types of HbO chambers. Multipatient HbO chambers have monitoring devices located within the chamber, while single-patient chambers have monitors located outside of the chamber with the cables passing through pressure-sealed port holes to attach to the patient.[33] Continuous pulse oximetry monitoring is less useful because of the high partial pressure of oxygen delivered. Invasive monitoring may be required for sicker patients. Because of the high fire risk associated with the high oxygen tensions, all monitors used in the chambers must be electrically safe and in compliance with National Fire Protection Association guidelines.[33]

Office-Based Anesthesia

Office-based anesthesia for dental, cosmetic, and maxillofacial procedures represents an emerging form of NORA. These locations are not subject to the same governmental regulations as the hospital and ambulatory surgery. Office-based anesthesia practices have minimal accreditation requirements.[34] The entire continuum of anesthesia and sedation may be performed in an office-based setting ranging from local anesthesia to general anesthesia. Office-based practices should be compliant with the same minimum monitoring standards, including pulse oximetry, capnography, ECG, NIBP, and temperature. Monitors and equipment for emergencies must be well maintained and functional.[34] The providers administering sedation in the office have to be able to evaluate the physical status and airway of the patient and select the candidates of office procedures appropriately.[35]

Intensive Care Unit

The number of procedures taking place in the intensive care unit setting has increased for various reasons. Intensivists may request support from the anesthesiologist due to the increased complexity of patients and procedures. Transportation of these patients to the operating room increases the risk of hemodynamic instability and poses significant morbidity and mortality. Anesthesia providers are increasingly expected to take care of critically ill patients in remote settings where few providers are familiar with the care sick patients. Preprocedural preparation is essential in this setting.

SUMMARY

The safe provision of NORA requires strict adherence to standardized monitoring guidelines. Basic monitoring for NORA should include pulse oximetry, capnography, ECG, and NIBP. Body temperature should also be measured in appropriate scenarios. High-risk anesthetics require advanced preparation and monitoring. Remote locations where complex procedures are performed on patients with ASA-PS of at least 3 must be equipped with appropriate monitoring capabilities.[36,37]

REFERENCES

1. Pino RM. The nature of anesthesia and procedural sedation outside of the operating room. Curr Opin Anaesthesiol 2007;20(4):347–51.
2. Lalwani K, Michel M. Pediatric sedation in North American children's hospitals: a survey of anesthesia providers. Paediatr Anaesth 2005;15(3):209–13.
3. Bhananker SM, Posner KL, Cheney FW, et al. Injury and liability associated with monitored anesthesia care: a closed claims analysis. Anesthesiology 2006; 104(2):228–34.
4. Metzner J, Posner KL, Domino KB. The risk and safety of anesthesia at remote locations: the US closed claims analysis. Curr Opin Anaesthesiol 2009;22(4): 502–8.
5. Caplan RA, Posner KL, Ward RJ, et al. Adverse respiratory events in anesthesia: a closed claims analysis. Anesthesiology 1990;72(5):828–33.
6. Tremper KK, Barker SJ. Pulse oximetry. Anesthesiology 1989;70(1):98–108.

7. Eichhorn JH. Pulse oximetry as a standard of practice in anesthesia. Anesthesiology 1993;78(3):423–6.
8. Severinghaus JW, Spellman MJ Jr. Pulse oximeter failure thresholds in hypotension and vasoconstriction. Anesthesiology 1990;73(3):532–7.
9. Krauss B, Hess DR. Capnography for procedural sedation and analgesia in the emergency department. Ann Emerg Med 2007;50(2):172–81.
10. Kannikeswaran N, Chen X, Sethuraman U. Utility of end tidal carbon dioxide monitoring in detection of hypoxia during sedation for brain magnetic resonance imaging in children with developmental disabilities. Paediatr Anaesth 2011; 21(12):1241–6.
11. Langhan ML, Chen L, Marshall C, et al. Detection of hypoventilation by capnography and its association with hypoxia in children undergoing sedation with ketamine. Pediatr Emerg Care 2011;27(5):394–7.
12. Green SM, Pershad J. Should capnographic monitoring be standard practice during emergency department procedural sedation and analgesia? Pro and con. Ann Emerg Med 2010;55(3):265–7.
13. Beitz A, Riphaus A, Meining A, et al. Capnographic monitoring reduces the incidence of arterial oxygen desaturation and hypoxemia during propofol sedation for colonoscopy: a randomized, controlled study (ColoCap Study). Am J Gastroenterol 2012;107(8):1205–12.
14. Deitch K, Miner J, Chudnofsky CR, et al. Does end tidal CO2 monitoring during emergency department procedural sedation and analgesia with propofol decrease the incidence of hypoxic events? A randomized, controlled trial. Ann Emerg Med 2010;55(3):258–64.
15. Stoelting RK, Miller RD. Basics of anesthesia. 5 edition. Philadelphia: Churchill Livingstone. The Elsevier; 2007.
16. Wax DB, Lin HM, Leibowitz AB. Invasive and concomitant noninvasive intraoperative blood pressure monitoring: observed differences in measurements and associated therapeutic interventions. Anesthesiology 2011;115(5):973–8.
17. Torossian A. Thermal management during anaesthesia and thermoregulation standards for the prevention of inadvertent perioperative hypothermia. Best Pract Res Clin Anaesthesiol 2008;22(4):659–68.
18. Missant C, Van de Velde M. Morbidity and mortality related to anaesthesia outside the operating room. Curr Opin Anaesthesiol 2004;17(4):323–7.
19. Frank SM, Beattie C, Christopherson R, et al. Unintentional hypothermia is associated with postoperative myocardial ischemia. The Perioperative Ischemia Randomized Anesthesia Trial Study Group. Anesthesiology 1993;78(3):468–76.
20. Kurz A, Sessler DI, Lenhardt R. Perioperative normothermia to reduce the incidence of surgical-wound infection and shorten hospitalization. Study of Wound Infection and Temperature Group. N Engl J Med 1996;334(19):1209–15.
21. Putzu M, Casati A, Berti M, et al. Clinical complications, monitoring and management of perioperative mild hypothermia: anesthesiological features. Acta Biomed 2007;78(3):163–9.
22. Kumar A, Anel R, Bunnell E, et al. Pulmonary artery occlusion pressure and central venous pressure fail to predict ventricular filling volume, cardiac performance, or the response to volume infusion in normal subjects. Crit Care Med 2004;32(3):691–9.
23. Boushel R, Langberg H, Olesen J, et al. Monitoring tissue oxygen availability with near infrared spectroscopy (NIRS) in health and disease. Scand J Med Sci Sports 2001;11(4):213–22.

24. Scott JP, Hoffman GM. Near-infrared spectroscopy: exposing the dark (venous) side of the circulation. Paediatr Anaesth 2014;24(1):74–88.
25. Mazzeo AT, Di Pasquale R, Settineri N, et al. Usefulness and limits of near infrared spectroscopy monitoring during endovascular neuroradiologic procedures. Minerva Anestesiol 2012;78(1):34–45.
26. Gamble C, Gamble J, Seal R, et al. Bispectral analysis during procedural sedation in the pediatric emergency department. Pediatr Emerg Care 2012;28(10): 1003–8.
27. Punjasawadwong Y, Phongchiewboon A, Bunchungmongkol N. Bispectral index for improving anaesthetic delivery and postoperative recovery. Cochrane Database Syst Rev 2014;(6):CD003843.
28. Patteson SK, Chesney JT. Anesthetic management for magnetic resonance imaging: problems and solutions. Anesth Analg 1992;74(1):121–8.
29. Taber KH, Thompson J, Coveler LA, et al. Invasive pressure monitoring of patients during magnetic resonance imaging. Can J Anaesth 1993;40(11):1092–5.
30. Saunders R, Erslon M, Vargo J. Modeling the costs and benefits of capnography monitoring during procedural sedation for gastrointestinal endoscopy. Endosc Int Open 2016;4(3):E340–51.
31. Robbertze R, Posner KL, Domino KB. Closed claims review of anesthesia for procedures outside the operating room. Curr Opin Anaesthesiol 2006;19(4):436–42.
32. Chakravarti SB, Mittnacht AJ, Katz JC, et al. Multisite near-infrared spectroscopy predicts elevated blood lactate level in children after cardiac surgery. J Cardiothorac Vasc Anesth 2009;23(5):663–7.
33. Weaver LK. Hyperbaric oxygen in the critically ill. Crit Care Med 2011;39(7): 1784–91.
34. Guidelines for office-based anesthesia [press release]. Approved by the ASA House of Delegates on October 13, 1999; last amended on October 21, 2009; and reaffirmed on October 15, 2014.
35. Petrocelli SR, Anderson JW, Hanks AR. DDT and dieldrin residues in selected biota from San Antonio Bay, Texas–1972. Pestic Monit J 1974;8(3):167–72.
36. Arato A. Physical properties of various cements used in orthodontics. SSO Schweiz Monatsschr Zahnheilkd 1974;84(5):535–58 [in German].
37. Metzner J, Domino KB. Risks of anesthesia or sedation outside the operating room: the role of the anesthesia care provider. Curr Opin Anaesthesiol 2010; 23(4):523–31.

Use of Anesthesiology Services in Radiology

Hansol Kim, MD[a,b], Jason Lane, MD, MPH[c],*, Rolf Schlichter, MD[d], Michael S. Stecker, MD[a,b], Richard Taus, MD[e]

KEYWORDS

- Non–operating room anesthesia (NORA) care • Interventional radiology
- Anesthesiology • Consultation • Communication • Collaboration

KEY POINTS

- Collaboration and close communication between the anesthesiologist and the interventional radiologist is critical to success of a non–operating room anesthesia (NORA) procedure.
- The preprocedural, intraprocedural, and postprocedural needs of patients may vary depending on the type of interventional procedure performed.
- In the era of increasing use of NORA care, anesthesiologists must become adept in providing support in remote, space-limited non–operating room suites.

INTRODUCTION

Technological advancements in imaging and intervention have allowed many disease processes to be treated outside of the operating room (OR). These advancements have provided alternative treatments to patients who are considered too high a risk or too unstable for traditional surgical procedures. As a result, there has been considerable increase in use of various levels of procedural sedation, including moderate procedural sedation (MPS), deep sedation or monitored anesthesia care (MAC), and general anesthesia (GA) in interventional radiology (IR) suites. From 2003 to 2008, a greater than 4-fold increase in use of MPS in interventional suites has been reported, including a parallel growth in MAC and GA cases.[1] Similarly, the anesthesiology community has also reported an overall increase in use of non–OR anesthesia (NORA) care

Disclosure Statement: No Disclosures.
[a] Department of Radiology, Division of Angiography and Interventional Radiology, Brigham and Women's Hospital, 75 Francis Street, Midcampus SR-340, Boston, MA 02115, USA; [b] Harvard Medical School, 25 Shattuck Street, Boston, MA 02115, USA; [c] Department of Anesthesiology, Vanderbilt University Medical Center, 1301 Medical Center Drive, 4648 TVC, Nashville, TN 37232, USA; [d] Hospital of the University of Pennsylvania, 6 Dulles, 3400 Spruce Street, Philadelphia, PA 19104, USA; [e] Morton Hospital, Taunton, MA, USA
* Corresponding author.
E-mail address: jason.lane@vanderbilt.edu

from 28.3% in 2010% to 35.9% in 2014.[2] It is projected that the number of NORA cases may approach or even exceed the number of traditional OR cases in the near future.[2] With this increase in the use of NORA services, there has been significant interest by the anesthesiology community to understand the specific needs and location-specific limitations of such procedures.

The main goal of this article is to review NORA services from the interventional radiologist's point of view. We address circumstances in which an anesthesiology evaluation may be requested, the expectations the interventional radiologist may have, and the types of limitations that may be encountered by the NORA practitioner. Understanding the intricacies of IR procedures by anesthesiologists is crucial to the success of the procedure and postprocedural care, and close communication and collaboration between the interventional radiologist and the anesthesiologist is critical for optimal patient outcome. Specific examples will be included in this review where applicable. Owing to completely different prioritization of needs and range of limitations, this paper does not address pediatric, neurologic, or cardiac interventional procedures. In addition, it does not address radiation-related concerns for anesthesiologists involved in such NORA procedures.

AMERICAN COLLEGE OF RADIOLOGY AND SOCIETY OF INTERVENTIONAL RADIOLOGY PRACTICE PARAMETER ON SEDATION AND ANALGESIA

In the setting of growing use of procedural sedation, the American College of Radiology (ACR) and Society of Interventional Radiology have put forth clinical practice guidelines pertaining to sedation and analgesia for practicing interventional radiologists based on the American Society of Anesthesiologists (ASA) physical status classification system.[3] In brief, patients under the ASA I (normal healthy patients) and ASA II (patients with mild systemic disease) categories are safe to proceed with MPS without the presence of anesthesiologists. However, there should be a low threshold for consultation with anesthesiology colleagues for intraprocedural sedation for patients under ASA III (patients with severe systemic disease) and ASA IV (patients with a constant threat to life) categories. Patients under ASA V category (moribund patient not expected to survive without procedure) should only be sedated by anesthesiologists.[3] Although most routinely performed outpatient procedures fall under ASA II and ASA III categories, and often do not require anesthesiologist care, all urgent inpatient procedures fall into ASA categories III through V, and availability of anesthesiologists may become critical for optimal patient outcome. It should be made clear that these parameters are meant to provide basic guidelines, and practicing interventional radiologists should practice good clinical judgment to determine analgesia and sedation needs of individual patients, taking into account patient-specific risk factors and procedural needs.

Often, patients are brought into the IR suite in an urgent or emergent setting for definitive treatment or as a temporary measure to stabilize and bridge them for surgery. Based on the ASA Closed Claims analysis, patients undergoing procedures outside of the OR were older (age >70 was 20% for NORA cases vs 12% for OR cases), sicker (69% of NORA cases being under ASA categories III–V vs 44% for OR cases), and more emergent (36% in NORA cases vs 15% for OR cases).[4] Furthermore, patients who have been deemed as nonsurgical candidates who are older and sicker are often referred to IR as a last effort to control disease. Other studies have reported similar findings, with an older mean age of NORA patients by 3.5 years compared with OR patients (95% CI, 3.5–3.5; $P<.001$), faster rate of annual increase in the mean age of NORA patients compared with OR patients

(P<.001), and a higher proportion of patients with ASA class III or V functional status in NORA patients compared with OR patients (37.6% vs 33.0%; P<.001) with statistically significant greater annual increase in ASA physical status in NORA patients (P<.001).[2] Based on this study, the median duration of NORA procedures was lower compared with OR cases (40 minutes vs 86 minutes; P<.001), however, more NORA cases occurred after normal working hours compared with surgery (16.7% vs 9.9%; P<.001).[2]

It should also be kept in mind that many IR procedures result in only mild, temporary discomfort and they may be performed under only the use of local anesthesia. However, when done on critically ill patients, even without any sedation, there may still be a need for intensive intraprocedural patient monitoring and concurrent treatment of underlying medical issues (eg, advanced airway management and suctioning in a patient with active hemoptysis undergoing bronchial artery embolization).

CONSIDERATIONS FOR ANESTHESIOLOGY CONSULTATION

Individual patient risk factors should be considered in determining whether MPS is appropriate, or if anesthesiologist consultation should be obtained.[3] Some of these risk factors are related to medical issues. One factor to be evaluated is a history of prior difficulties with anesthesia or MPS. Airway abnormalities such as obstructive sleep apnea, tracheal stenosis, and facial dysmorphism should be considered. Comorbid conditions including respiratory disease, cardiovascular disease (including critical aortic stenosis and congestive heart failure), and symptomatic gastroesophageal reflux should also be taken into account. Systemic issues including recent sedation or anesthesia, a catastrophic event within 24 to 48 hours of the planned procedure, presence of sepsis, hemodynamic instability, and the potential for polypharmacy should also be reviewed.

Anesthesiologist evaluation may also be necessary if it is deemed that the patient will not be able to cooperate with intraprocedural instructions (eg, following instructions for breath-holds) in the setting of altered mental status or a significant language barrier.

In the setting of critical illness and opioid tolerance, such as oncologic patients who are in need of large amounts of medications for baseline pain control, evaluation of their chronic pain regimen is critical, because safe levels of MPS may not result in adequate sedation and analgesia. In such cases, consultation with anesthesiology and the pain service would be ideal to optimize intraprocedural sedation, as well as postprocedural analgesia.

When patients are referred to interventional radiologists for consultation in anticipation of an elective procedure, they can then be referred for outpatient anesthesia evaluation and clearance. In fact, the proportion of outpatient NORA cases has increased from 69.7% in 2010% to 73.3% in 2014 (P<.001).[2] When patients have risk factors and comorbidities as those described, it is preferred to schedule a procedure with anesthesiology support, as opposed to needing to reschedule the procedure with anesthesiology after a failed attempt, or requiring a stat anesthesiology consultation or intervention while the patient is on the table in distress.[1]

The use of MAC or GA may also be specifically requested by the patient, especially in the setting of significant concern or anxiety for the procedure, or in the setting of claustrophobia if the procedure is planned in a computed tomography (CT) or magnetic resonance (MR) scanner. However, sometimes education and reassurance by an anesthesiologist can help the patient to be more comfortable with MPS when otherwise appropriate.

Procedure-specific patient issues should also be considered. For example, with transarterial chemoembolization of hepatic metastasis in the setting of carcinoid tumor, there can be a marked release of serotonin resulting in carcinoid crisis with concomitant flushing, bronchoconstriction, nausea/vomiting, significant abdominal pain, and secondary restrictive cardiomyopathy. Similarly, percutaneous ablation of adrenal metastasis (and of adjacent normal adrenal gland) may result in release of catecholamines, with resultant hypertensive crisis, cardiac irritability, arrhythmias, and troponin leak.[5] In this case, the type of ablation also affects the timing of catecholamine surge; heat-based radiofrequency and microwave ablations result in a catecholamine surge at the time of burning, whereas cryoablation results in a surge during the thawing of the ice ball.[1] Pretreatment strategies have not been shown to necessarily inhibit a catecholamine surge.[1] Central venous percutaneous transluminal stent placement in setting of malignant superior vena cava syndrome also poses a unique high risk for airway compromise, because the airway is also frequently involved with tumor and obstructs more easily in the supine position after sedation is administered.

Most patients requiring MAC or GA are severely ill, with ASA physical status III and higher, but when a procedure is emergent, there may not be sufficient time to do thorough evaluation or optimization before the procedure. In fact, about 70% of IR procedures are scheduled less than 48 hours in advance.[1] In the setting of emergent transjugular portosystemic shunt (TIPS) or angiography and embolization for upper or lower gastrointestinal hemorrhage, traumatic splenic, hepatic, or pelvic bleeds, and other instances of active acute hemorrhage, patients often need to be called to the IR suite before their low hemoglobin/hematocrit or coagulopathy can be completely stabilized or reversed. The anesthesiologist must then become part of the process of optimization of the patient during the procedure, just as in OR cases for trauma.

USE TRENDS AND PROCEDURAL NEEDS

In the day-to-day practice of IR, one observes that there is a general belief by referring physicians that, because IR procedures are less invasive than traditional surgery, that they are easier and lower risk. However, procedures such as TIPS, thrombolysis, and embolization can be technically challenging and can have the potential for major morbidity, particularly when performed emergently in patients who cannot be fully optimized. Based on the ASA Closed Claims database, death was a more common adverse event for NORA cases compared with OR cases (54% of complications vs 29%; $P<.001$).[4] Although that group attributed the higher reported claims for death in NORA cases to remote location as primary source of risk for patients with resultant oversedation, inadequate oxygenation, and inadequate ventilation during MAC, it is likely multifactorial, with procedural risk, an older and less healthy patient population, and more emergent procedure contributing to mortality. In addition, the frequency of NORA cases has been reported to be 1.7 times greater after routine work hours compared with OR cases, presenting additional risk from less familiarity with the work area and further limitations in resources and staff.[2]

There are wide variations on the preferred level of sedation for different procedures based on institutional practice, availability of anesthesiologists, patient factors, and interventional radiologist preference. Several trends are clear in the United States and Europe. The use of MAC and GA are favored for TIPS and nephrolithotomy.[6,7] In addition, there has been a tendency for use for percutaneous nephrostomy, ureteral stricture dilatation, biliary drain placement, biliary stricture dilatation and stent placement, cholecystostomy, gastrostomy and jejunostomy, and embolization procedures.[6,7] Further, these studies are from the late 1990s, and with increasingly more complex interventional procedures performed on even more morbid patients, we suspect use of MAC and GA has become even more critical in the practice of IR.

What do these procedures have in common? TIPS, nephrolithotomy, and complex embolization procedures often require prolonged sedation, prolonged ability to stay still, and may be associated with significant intraprocedural and postprocedural pain. TIPS procedures are often performed in sick, hemodynamically unstable patients, and concomitant intraprocedural optimization of the patient by means of massive blood transfusions may be taking place in setting of massive upper gastrointestinal hemorrhage. The anesthesia team is better able to manage acute fluid shifts that may have dire outcome compared with the primary operator, who is actively focused on the technical aspects of a challenging procedure and trying to control the bleeding.

In the setting of septic shock from obstructive uropathy, vasoconstrictors may be required and restrict the use of MPS owing to further decreases in blood pressure from the use of such agents. This consideration in turn may reduce the ability to appropriately sedate and provide analgesia to the patient.

The ability of the patient to hold their breath becomes critical in biliary and urinary drainage procedures, especially while trying to access a nondilated system. To optimally visualize the organ of interest with imaging, reliably deploy embolization agents or stents, and reduce complications, the ability of the patient to stay still becomes critical, because motion can result in nontarget embolization or stent maldeployment.

Among the various interventional procedures, biliary procedures have been shown to be associated with the highest rates of adverse events with MPS, including statistically significant total adverse and respiratory events.[8] This trend is thought to be due to the use of higher doses of sedatives and analgesics to achieve an appropriate level of analgesia and prolonged sedation time.[8] Therefore, continuous monitoring of patient's ventilation status with continuous capnography is critical and, when appropriate, timely anesthesia support may be needed.

With regard to intraprocedural patient positioning, age and body mass index also play a role in determining the type of sedation.[9] Patients may not be able to tolerate prone positioning with MPS or MAC, such as for percutaneous nephrostomy placement, translumbar endoleak embolization, and translumbar venous catheter placement.

UNDERSTANDING THE INTRICACIES OF INTERVENTIONAL RADIOLOGY PROCEDURES AND THE INTERVENTIONAL RADIOLOGY SUITE

Understanding the specifics of IR procedures is critical for all phases of procedural care. In cases of CT- or MR-guided procedures where the patient is physically moved into and out of the bore of the imaging device, positioning of the patient with respect to length of intravenous tubing, endotracheal ventilation tubing, monitor leads and cords, and the potential for sterile field contamination, planning is vital before the procedure even starts. As mentioned, the potential for carcinoid syndrome or catecholamine surge must be anticipated and planned for. Additionally, understanding the reasoning and timing behind when breath holds are required and when paralytics might be required will help to reduce procedural time.

Unlike the OR, where the recommended ambient temperature range is between 68°F and 75°F, based on infection prevention and engineer requirements,[10] angiography systems, ultrasound, CT, and MR scanners require strict equipment temperature control owing to the heat they produce themselves, with tolerance of angiography system equipment optimized at 68°F.[1] When imaging equipment overheats, it can result in unexpected termination of a procedure or require that the patient be moved to another suite. Therefore, strict environmental temperature control, patient temperature monitoring, and support with devices such as Bair Huggers (Arizant Healthcare Inc., Eden Prairie, MN) must be used to maintain optimal equipment and patient body temperatures.[1]

Procedures performed in an MR interventional suite have their own special precautions. Strict regulations, standards, guidelines, and recommendations are in place by governing bodies such as the American College of Radiology, and are briefly summarized here.[11] All operators, personnel, and patients should undergo thorough review and fill out a checklist to assess the for presence of ferrous material, including but not limited to pacemakers and defibrillators, surgical clips, cochlear implants, and implantable pain pumps or insulin pumps.[12] Dermal anesthetic patches containing ferrous material and coiled wires may induce skin burns, and should be removed or repositioned before the start of the procedure.[11] Also, it must be recognized that the magnetic field may alter electrocardiographic data. Only equipment deemed MR compatible or MR safe should enter the MR environment with certain restrictions, including the anesthesia machine and cart, electrocardiograph leads, wires, and tubing. With a giant magnet as its basis, non-MR safe stretchers, oxygen tanks, and intravenous line poles can easily become fatal projectiles when brought across the threshold of an MR. Earplugs should also be provided to the patient and those remaining in the MR suite, because hearing injury may occur with repeated exposure to loud noise from the MR machine.[12] In the setting of an emergency, where a patient needs cardiopulmonary resuscitation, basic maneuvers, including protection of the airway, ventilation, and chest compressions, may be initiated by staff already in, or cleared to be in, the MR scanner. However, the patient should be immediately moved out of the magnet into a predesignated MR-safe location for subsequent treatment.[11] The MR technologist and interventional radiologist may serve as excellent resources for anesthesiologists not familiar with MR environment and safety.

COMMUNICATION AND COLLABORATION FOR PROCEDURE PLANNING

If a patient is considered too high risk to proceed with MPS, consultation with anesthesiologists will be arranged to provide intraprocedural sedation and analgesia. In such cases, a few options may exist, including regional anesthesia, MAC, and GA with or without paralysis. Regional anesthesia, although frequently used in the obstetric OR, has not been widely used in IR procedures, partly owing to difficulty in applicability. For example, patients who are undergoing thrombectomy and thrombolysis, with subsequent need for prolonged anticoagulation, will be placed at a greater than necessary risk of bleeding in the epidural space, compared with alternatives such as MAC or GA.

Close communication and collaboration between the anesthesiologist and the interventional radiologist is critical for optimal patient outcome. Because not all patients and IR procedures are created equal, creative adaptation of techniques may be required to achieve the therapeutic goal. Therefore, the anesthesiologist and interventional radiologist must be in continuous communication to successfully complete the intended procedure as efficiently and safely as possible. Direct and open communication also allows anesthesiologists to administer booster analgesia during more painful aspects of a procedure, such as during tract dilatation, drainage tube insertion, angioplasty balloon inflation, or tumor ablation.

Before the start of the procedure, the interventional radiologist must discuss with the anesthesia team the positioning of the patient, the operators, and the equipment to determine optimal anesthesiology equipment set up. Because the anesthesia machine and equipment cart compete for space with the rest of the imaging equipment and supplies, preprocedural planning of the placement of such equipment and patient may reduce procedural time and allow more optimal access to the airway.[12] The more familiar the anesthesiologist is with basic IR procedures, the better and more meaningful this communication will be. Additionally, digital subtraction angiography, CT, or MR image acquisitions may require all operators, including the anesthesiologist, to temporarily step out of the interventional suite. The ability to monitor the patient's vital signs through a window, via a camera, or on an additional monitor, may be critical.[12]

The ideal time to discuss the needs and expectations of the procedure may be during scheduled IR morning rounds (if available at one's institution) or alternatively at the time of preprocedural time out.[13] Participation of anesthesiologists during IR morning rounds allows both teams to discuss their needs ahead of time to improve procedural efficiency and room set up and turnover, and also allows the sorting out of any unexpected issues. This practice also creates a sense of team camaraderie, allowing collaborative contribution of both teams' expertise to successfully treat patients. Although this may be a common practice in academic institutions, anesthesiologists may not be widely available in the community hospital setting for morning rounds. In the era of rising NORA cases as well as a nationwide push for efficiency, the adaptation of such practices may be warranted to provide optimal patient care.

Anesthesiologists should feel comfortable working in the IR procedure suite; the American College of Radiology/Society of Interventional Radiology guidelines recommend that all IR suites provide a continuous oxygen supply with backup, airway equipment, a continuous suction apparatus, and emergency medications, as well as equipment such as a defibrillator, monitors with visible and audible output for pulse oximetry, blood pressure cuff, multilead electrocardiographic monitor, a means of monitoring ventilation, and capnography. Also recommended is the availability of a stethoscope, phone or other 2-way communication device, emergent light source, and emergent electric power.[3] Because IR procedure suites are often located remotely from the OR, all anesthetics, reversal agents, and other medications commonly available to the anesthesiologist in the OR should be made available in a nearby medication dispensing system. However, such guidelines have not been in place for long; older IR suites may not provide such equipment and may have significant space restrictions. Practicing anesthesiologists should become familiar with individual institution's limitations and plan procedures accordingly.

Although controversial, patients with baseline renal insufficiency are at increased risk for contrast-induced nephropathy after the administration of intravenous radiographic contrast. Provision of intravenous hydration, preprocedure, intraprocedure, and postprocedure can help to mitigate this risk.

The decision to paralyze the patient should ideally be made ahead of time during preprocedural planning, collaboratively between the anesthesiologist and the interventional radiologist. If procedural needs change over time, the operator should communicate this to the anesthesiologist as soon as possible. The risks and benefits, as well as the potential effect on room turnover by use of paralytics, should be considered. Typically, complex embolization procedures and multilevel vertebral augmentation require complete paralysis of the patient.

In the event a patient acutely decompensates and is in need of additional intravenous or intraarterial access for resuscitation and/or further monitoring, the expertise of the interventional radiologist may be extremely helpful in placing such lines. However, because the initial reaction for the interventionalist may be to step away to provide room for the anesthesiology team to work, it is necessary to directly communicate the needs of the anesthesiology team to the IR team.

Because more NORA cases are occurring during off-hours, compared with surgery, with less availability of support staff, additional equipment, and help from colleagues and direct communication with rest of the on-call staff and colleagues should be established and a system to provide assistance must be in place.[12] In contrast, at institutions with limited availability of anesthesiologists, an interventional radiologist may need to proceed with an emergent procedure under MPS, or even just local anesthesia, if a delay in the procedure is believed to have a high probability of resulting in a fatal outcome.

POSTPROCEDURE CARE

After the IR procedure, patients may be sent directly back to the inpatient floor, or first observed in the IR recovery room or in the postanesthesia care unit for several hours before transport to the inpatient floor or discharge home, depending on the patient and procedural circumstances. During this time, the patient is observed for the development of procedure-related complications, such as bleeding at an access site, signs of end-organ ischemia, evidence of a precipitated systemic infection, or ablation-related myoglobinemia. Because each IR procedure comes with specific complication risks, expected outcomes, laboratory findings, and management issues, including medications to avoid, this information should be closely communicated between the interventional radiologist and the anesthesiologist who will be recovering the patient.

Some patients may require indwelling catheters to be left overnight with continuous anticoagulant and/or thrombolytic infusions, such as heparin and alteplase, and early communication and planning for the use of such items can ensure that such medications and intensive care unit beds for monitoring are readily available before or by the end of the procedure.[9]

Although lactated Ringer's solution is often used in postoperative patients, it should generally be avoided in IR patients after ablations or end-organ embolization, because lactated Ringer's solution contains potassium chloride, and subsequent hyperkalemia may ensue. If the patient develops significant myoglobinemia, treatment with adequate hydration with or without sodium bicarbonate may be warranted.

A catecholamine surge after adrenal metastasis ablation may require close cardiac monitoring, as well as antihypertensive and antiarrhythmic medications.

FUTURE AREAS FOR IMPROVEMENT

Because only a certain number of angiography suites, ultrasound, CT, and MR rooms are available for procedures in a given day, efficient room turnover is crucial to meet the day-to-day requirements of a busy IR service. Typically, MPS is preferred by practicing interventional radiologists for most procedures owing to its ease and fast room turnover. MPS avoids room downtime for anesthesia set up, preprocedural intubation, and postprocedural extubation or recovery.[6,7] Unlike the main OR, where anesthesia cases are constantly tracked and updated, an equivalent system of interdepartmental communication and patient tracking for NORA cases may not be available.[1] As NORA cases continue to expand, development of such systems may be of tremendous value.

Because more NORA cases occur during off hours as compared with surgery,[2] wide availability of anesthesiologists on call for such urgent and emergent procedures is very important. In addition, these patients will generally have more comorbidities and may not be able to be optimized fully. All efforts and resources should be used to avoid placing a critically ill patient at a higher risk by performing an IR procedure under MPS owing to unavailability of an anesthesiologist.

Typically, both IR and anesthesiology teams work with limited resources and staff during off hours. Although a single interventional radiologist, assistant, radiologic technologist, nurse, and anesthesiologist may be sufficient for most procedures, there may be times when additional help is needed, especially in the setting of multiple traumatic injuries. In such cases, both teams should have programs in place where additional personnel can be called in to help with multiple concurrent procedures.

There is a wide variability in availability of anesthesiologists for interventional procedures in academic and community care centers. Although many academic institutions with high NORA volume are likely to have regularly scheduled blocks of time with anesthesiologists or even a separate NORA team, community centers may not. Thus, they may have a difficult time receiving anesthesia support for ASA physical status III to V patients. Many interventional radiologists in the community setting may have to schedule their NORA cases on both the IR schedule and the OR schedule, which introduces the possibility of errors. Nationwide efforts to standardize NORA availability, interventional suite set up, and communication between anesthesiologist and interventionalists may help to provide the most efficient and safe care the patient deserves.

REFERENCES

1. Schenker MP, Martin R, Shyn PB, et al. Interventional radiology and anesthesia. Anesthesiol Clin 2009;27:87–94.
2. Nagrebetsky A, Gabriel RA, Dutton RP, et al. Growth of nonoperating room anesthesia care in the United States: a contemporary trends analysis. Anesth Analg 2017;124(4):1261–7.
3. American College of Radiology (ACR). ACR-SIR practice parameter for sedation/analgesia, resolution 23, 2015. Available at: https://www.acr.org/~/media/F194CBB800AB43048B997A75938AB482.pdf. Accessed March 11, 2017.
4. Metzner J, Posner KL, Domino KB. The risk and safety of anesthesia at remote locations: the US closed claims analysis. Curr Opin Anaesthesiol 2009;22:502–8.
5. Fintelmann FJ, Tuncali K, Puchner S, et al. Catecholamine surge during image guided ablation of adrenal gland metastases: predictors, consequences, and recommendations for management. J Vasc Interv Radiol 2016;27(3):395–402.
6. Haslam PJ, Yap B, Mueller PR, et al. Anesthesia practice and clinical trends in interventional radiology: a European survey. Cardiovasc Intervent Radiol 2000;23:256–61.
7. Mueller PR, Wittenberg KH, Kaufman JA, et al. Patterns of anesthesia and nursing care for interventional radiology procedures: a national survey of physician practices and preferences. Radiology 1997;202:339–43.
8. Arepally A, Oeschsle D, Kirkwood S, et al. Safety of conscious sedation in interventional radiology. Cardiovasc Intervent Radiol 2001;24(3):185–90.
9. Rafiei P, Walser EM, Duncan JR, et al. Society of interventional radiology IR preprocedure patient safety checklist by the safety and health committee. J Vasc Interv Radiol 2016;27(5):695–9.

10. Association of perioperative registered nurses. Guidelines for a safe environment of care, part 2. In: Guidelines for perioperative practice 2015. Available at: https://www.aorn.org/guidelines/clinical-resources/clinical-faqs/environment-of-care. Accessed March 11, 2017.

11. Kanal E, Barkovich AJ, Bell C, et al. ACR guidance document for safe MR practices: 2007. AJR Am J Roentgenol 2007;188:1447–74.

12. Cutter TW. Radiologists and anesthesiologists. Anesthesiol Clin 2009;27(1): 95–106.

13. Angle JF, Nemcek AA, Cohen AM, et al. Quality improvement guidelines for preventing wrong site, wrong procedure, and wrong person errors: application of the joint commission "universal protocol for preventing wrong site, wrong procedure, wrong person surgery" to the practice of interventional radiology. J Vasc Interv Radiol 2008;19(8):1145–51.

An Anesthesiologist's View of Tumor Ablation in the Radiology Suite

Annie Amin, MD[a], Jason Lane, MD, MPH[b],*,
Thomas Cutter, MD, MAEd[a]

KEYWORDS

- Non-operating room anesthesia (NORA) care • Collaboration • Tumor ablation
- Interventional radiology • Anesthesiology

KEY POINTS

- Novel tumor ablation techniques have revolutionized the approach to treating solid organ tumors.
- Various forms of energy (cold, heat, radio wave, and laser) are applied to tumors using different imaging modalities.
- Image-guided tumor ablation procedures have created a new paradigm for treating tumors in patients who otherwise would not tolerate a traditional open procedure.
- Knowledge of these various ablation technologies and procedures by an anesthesiologist is critical to patient safety and optimal outcome.

INTRODUCTION

Tumor ablation is the direct application of chemical-based or energy-based therapies to eradicate or substantially destroy focal tumors.[1] Chemical ablation is a non–energy-based therapy using chemotherapeutic agents (chemoembolization), ethanol, or acetic acid. Energy-based therapies are thermal or nonthermal and include radiofrequency ablation (RFA), cryoablation, and irreversible electroporation (IRE). Tumor ablation is performed for curative, palliative, or debulking purposes. Ablative therapies often require image guidance for precise needle, probe, or catheter placement and use fluoroscopy, CT, MRI, or ultrasound. If anesthesia assistance is requested for ablation procedures, the anesthesiologist must be aware of the specific safety concerns and anesthetic considerations for each type of ablation therapy as well as the

Disclosure Statement: No disclosures.
[a] Department of Anesthesiology, University of Chicago, 5841 South Maryland Avenue, Chicago, IL 60637, USA; [b] Department of Anesthesiology, Vanderbilt University Medical Center, 1301 Medical Center Drive, 4648 TVC, Nashville, TN 37232, USA
* Corresponding author.
E-mail address: jason.lane@vanderbilt.edu

imaging modality. Thermal therapies require precautions to prevent trauma to surrounding healthy tissue from high temperatures. IRE has numerous anesthetic implications, including monitoring for procedure-related ventricular arrhythmias.

Anesthesiologists must maintain safe practices in the non–operating room anesthesia environment. Ultrasound, used alone, does not require additional safety strategies, but fluoroscopy and CT necessitate strategies to mitigate exposure to ionizing radiation. For MRI procedures, the importance of preventing ferrous materials and equipment from harming patients and staff is paramount. The preanesthesia evaluation should be conducted with these modality-specific concerns in mind.

CHEMICAL ABLATION

During chemical ablation, agents, such as ethanol or acetic acid, induce tumor cell death and coagulation necrosis.[1] The benefits of chemical ablation are low cost and simple technique. Success destroying large solid tumors is limited by poor and nonuniform diffusion, so chemical ablation is typically used as adjuvant therapy.[2] Ethanol ablation treats benign thyroid, thyroglossal, and renal cysts and often yields favorable outcomes after multiple treatment sessions.[3–5] Chemical ablation procedures are typically performed with local anesthesia and do not require an anesthesiologist.

Chemoembolization is currently limited to hepatic tumors, either primary or metastatic. A catheter is inserted into the femoral artery and guided under fluoroscopy into the hepatic artery where contrast material is injected to identify the arterial supply to the tumor. A chemotherapeutic agent (eg, doxorubicin) is then injected and is followed by an embolic agent (eg, iodized poppy seed oil). The latter limits the tumor's blood supply and traps the chemotherapeutic agent in close proximity to the tumor. Combination therapy with cisplatin, doxorubicin, and mitomycin C enhances the tumor-specific toxicity.[6] The procedure is typically performed without an anesthesiologist. If anesthesia is requested, the primary anesthetic concerns are patient comorbidities, coagulopathies, and hepatic insufficiency.

RADIOFREQUENCY ABLATION

RFA is an energy-based thermal therapy that typically targets kidney, lung, breast, bone, and liver tumors. It offers an alternative for patients who may not be candidates for surgical resection because of size, location, poor organ function reserve, or comorbidities. It also may be combined with partial surgical resection for tumors not amenable to complete resection. Because healthy tissue is better able to withstand heat, radiofrequency energy preferentially destroys the tumor and only a small edge of normal tissue around its perimeter. The heat also cauterizes small blood vessels and reduces the risk of bleeding. Ablation can be performed percutaneously or directly within the tumor via laparoscopy or laparotomy with the assistance of CT, ultrasound, or PET.[7,8] Most radiofrequency devices use a single monopolar electrode and disperse the current through 1 or more grounding pads.

The least invasive approach is percutaneous. Complications have been reported and include third-degree burns of the abdominal wall from the tract-ablation portion of the procedure, abscess formation from bile duct injury, postprocedure myocardial infarction, and heat necrosis of the diaphragm resulting in sepsis and death.[8] Because the process produces heat, precautions must be taken when the electrode is adjacent to critical structures. As an example, when RFA was applied to a mediastinal lymph node, a temperature probe was placed at the endotracheal tube cuff to monitor the tracheal temperature. When the temperature rose, chilled saline was substituted for air in the cuff to prevent tracheal trauma.[9]

The anesthetic technique is dictated by the procedure and patient comorbidities. Moderate sedation is often adequate for a percutaneous approach,[10] but for patients who experience severe anxiety and pain, general anesthesia may be warranted. General anesthesia during RFA may provide numerous benefits, among them higher-power settings, longer RFA times, and less respiratory motion artifact during tumor mapping and probe placement.[11,12] Pain during conscious sedation or epidural anesthesia may be managed by lowering power settings, but this may lead to incomplete tumor ablation and increased potential for recurrence.[13] After epidural anesthesia, supplemental intravenous opioids may be needed for referred pain.

Anesthesiologists also should be aware of postprocedure complications. Post–tumor ablation syndrome is a not uncommon condition that manifests as a flulike illness with fever, malaise, myalgias, pain at the ablation site, nausea, and vomiting. It typically presents within 48 hours and is self-limiting with complete resolution in 7 days to 10 days. Symptoms may be more severe in patients who have ablation of liver lesions.[14] If symptoms persist, clinicians should be concerned about concurrent infections, such as a liver abscess, intestinal perforation with peritonitis, infected pleural effusion, and pneumonia.[15,16]

CRYOABLATION

Cryoablation is used for tumors in the lung, liver, breast, kidney, or prostate. Liquid nitrogen or gaseous argon destroys tissue by direct freezing, denaturation of cellular proteins, cell rupture, cell dehydration, and ischemia. Patient comfort and safety are provided with local or general anesthesia.[17] Cryoablation offers intrinsic pain relief because of the cooling effect on nerves (cryoanalgesia) and may require less sedation than thermal ablation therapies.[18,19] Concerns include inflammation and associated problems from the thawing phase after lung cryoablation or hemorrhage from the cracking of a cryoablated liver.[6]

IRREVERSIBLE ELECTROPORATION

IRE using CT for localization is a new nonthermal technique for tumor ablation. It uses pulsating electric current to induce changes in a cell membrane resulting in apoptosis.[1] Unlike thermal ablation, there is no heat sink effect, where heat is lost due to the cool flow of adjacent blood vessels,[20] and there is less risk of injury to surrounding tissue. IRE has been used to treat liver, kidney, and lung tumors.

The electrical impulses in IRE cause direct muscle stimulation necessitating muscle relaxation throughout the procedure. Ventricular arrhythmias with hemodynamic instability have been reported, so a 5-lead ECG and arterial cannulation for blood pressure monitoring are prudent. Use of a synchronizer to time the impulses with the ECG tracing may minimize the risk of arrhythmias.[21] Depending on the location of the tumor, positioning for the CT scan for optimal imaging of the tumor may require that the patient extend the arms above the head, so care must be taken to prevent brachial plexus injuries. Patients with a large tumor burden or preexisting renal dysfunction are at risk for electrolyte disturbances, and their blood chemistry should be monitored frequently. Given its complexity, the procedure must be performed with patients under general anesthesia. Postprocedure pain is generally mild and treated with intermittent opioids. Other sequalae are typically benign, but pneumothoraces, hematoma formation, transient transaminitis, portal vein, and bile duct strictures have been reported.[21,22]

MRI-GUIDED NEUROSURGICAL ABLATION WITH LASER DIODE (LASER INTERSTITIAL THERMAL THERAPY) FOR EPILEPSY AND BRAIN TUMORS

With the advent of image-guided tumor ablation in radiology, various surgical disciplines are beginning to treat tumors via these minimally invasive approaches using novel ablation techniques outside the normal confines of the operating room. Neurosurgeons are beginning to treat brain tumors and epilepsy with an MRI-guided laser ablation technique. These procedures typically start in the operating room with a small 1-cm bur hole made in the skull over the tumor. Then using a combination of hardware and software, a disposable laser probe is carefully advanced to the center of the brain tumor or epileptogenic focus. The patient is then brought to the MRI scanner while still under general endotracheal anesthesia, with the laser probe in place. In the MRI scanner, the targeted lesion in the brain is ablated using laser interstitial thermal therapy[23] and dose monitoring via MRI thermometry. This technique allows for precise ablation of brain lesions of varying sizes and shapes, in a wide variety of locations. Typically patients are discharged to home next day.

SUMMARY

As invasive techniques in radiology suites become more common, the need for anesthesia support will increase. Preprocedural anesthesia care is similar to that provided for patients in an operating room. The additional requirements and constraints of the imaging environment and the procedure are unique and require specific awareness and strategies. Just as in the operating room, there is frequently no single best anesthetic technique for a given procedure. The anesthetic should be aligned with the demands of the procedure and the skill sets of the providers. Patient safety always takes precedence, and the location should never be permitted to compromise care.

Radiologists serve a critical function, deciding whether to consult an anesthesiologist or perform a procedure alone. If the decision is to proceed with moderate sedation administered by a nonanesthesia professional, the importance of vigilant clinical monitoring cannot be overstated. In all cases, patients deserve care that is consistent with the parameters, guidelines, and standards established by the various accrediting agencies and professional societies. There should be no exceptions.

REFERENCES

1. Ahmed M, Solbiati L, Brace CL, et al. Image-guided tumor ablation: standardization of terminology and reporting criteria–a 10-year update. J Vasc Interv Radiol 2014;25(11):1691–705.e1694.
2. Ahmed M, Brace CL, Lee FT Jr, et al. Principles of and advances in percutaneous ablation. Radiology 2011;258(2):351–69.
3. Reverter JL, Alonso N, Avila M, et al. Evaluation of efficacy, safety, pain perception and health-related quality of life of percutaneous ethanol injection as first-line treatment in symptomatic thyroid cysts. BMC Endocr Disord 2015;15:73.
4. Lee DK, Seo JW, Park HS, et al. Efficacy of ethanol ablation for thyroglossal duct cyst. Ann Otol Rhinol Laryngol 2015;124(1):62–7.
5. Singh I, Mehrotra G. Selective ablation of symptomatic dominant renal cysts using 99% ethanol in adult polycystic kidney disease. Urology 2006;68(3):482–7 [discussion: 487–8].
6. Leyendecker JR, Dodd GD 3rd. Minimally invasive techniques for the treatment of liver tumors. Semin Liver Dis 2001;21(2):283–91.

7. Shyn PB, Tremblay-Paquet S, Palmer K, et al. Breath-hold PET/CT-guided tumour ablation under general anaesthesia: accuracy of tumour image registration and projected ablation zone overlap. Clin Radiol 2017;72(3):223–9.
8. Wood TF, Rose DM, Chung M, et al. Radiofrequency ablation of 231 unresectable hepatic tumors: indications, limitations, and complications. Ann Surg Oncol 2000; 7(8):593–600.
9. Hanazaki M, Taga N, Nakatsuka H, et al. Anesthetic management of radiofrequency ablation of mediastinal metastatic lymph nodes adjacent to the trachea. Anesth Analg 2006;103(4):1041–2.
10. McGhana JP, Dodd GD 3rd. Radiofrequency ablation of the liver: current status. AJR Am J Roentgenol 2001;176(1):3–16.
11. Kettenbach J, Kostler W, Rucklinger E, et al. Percutaneous saline-enhanced radiofrequency ablation of unresectable hepatic tumors: initial experience in 26 patients. AJR Am J Roentgenol 2003;180(6):1537–45.
12. Gupta A, Raman JD, Leveillee RJ, et al. General anesthesia and contrast-enhanced computed tomography to optimize renal percutaneous radiofrequency ablation: multi-institutional intermediate-term results. J Endourol 2009;23(7): 1099–105.
13. Kuo YH, Chung KC, Hung CH, et al. The impact of general anesthesia on radiofrequency ablation of hepatocellular carcinoma. Kaohsiung J Med Sci 2014; 30(11):559–65.
14. Wah TM, Arellano RS, Gervais DA, et al. Image-guided percutaneous radiofrequency ablation and incidence of post-radiofrequency ablation syndrome: prospective survey. Radiology 2005;237(3):1097–102.
15. Zagoria RJ, Chen MY, Shen P, et al. Complications from radiofrequency ablation of liver metastases. Am Surg 2002;68(2):204–9.
16. Livraghi T, Solbiati L, Meloni MF, et al. Treatment of focal liver tumors with percutaneous radio-frequency ablation: complications encountered in a multicenter study. Radiology 2003;226(2):441–51.
17. Shingleton WB, Sewell PE Jr. Percutaneous renal tumor cryoablation with magnetic resonance imaging guidance. J Urol 2001;165(3):773–6.
18. Trescot AM. Cryoanalgesia in interventional pain management. Pain Physician 2003;6(3):345–60.
19. Truesdale CM, Soulen MC, Clark TW, et al. Percutaneous computed tomography-guided renal mass radiofrequency ablation versus cryoablation: doses of sedation medication used. J Vasc Interv Radiol 2013;24(3):347–50.
20. Pillai K, Akhter J, Chua TC, et al. Heat sink effect on tumor ablation characteristics as observed in monopolar radiofrequency, bipolar radiofrequency, and microwave, using ex vivo calf liver model. Medicine (Baltimore) 2015;94(9):e580.
21. Ball C, Thomson KR, Kavnoudias H. Irreversible electroporation: a new challenge in "out of operating theater" anesthesia. Anesth Analg 2010;110(5):1305–9.
22. Fruhling P, Nilsson A, Duraj F, et al. Single-center nonrandomized clinical trial to assess the safety and efficacy of irreversible electroporation (IRE) ablation of liver tumors in humans: Short to mid-term results. Eur J Surg Oncol 2017;43(4):751–7.
23. Medvid R, Ruiz A, Komotar RJ, et al. Current applications of MRI-guided laser interstitial thermal therapy in the treatment of brain neoplasms and epilepsy: a radiologic and neurosurgical overview. AJNR Am J Neuroradiol 2015;36(11): 1998–2006.

A Radiologist's View of Tumor Ablation in the Radiology Suite

Sharath K. Bhagavatula, MD[a], Jason Lane, MD, MPH[b],*,
Paul Shyn, MD[a]

KEYWORDS

- Tumor ablation • Non–operating room anesthesia (NORA) care
- Interventional radiology • Anesthesiology • Collaboration

KEY POINTS

- There are a wide variety of tumor ablation techniques (eg, radiofrequency ablation, microwave ablation, and cryoablation) now available to treat tumors in a wide variety of locations in the body.
- Image guidance (eg, ultrasound, CT, MRI) allows interventional radiologists to target and treat tumors in a safe and effective manner.
- Collaboration and communication between the anesthesiologist and radiologist is critical to safe and successful tumor ablation in the radiology suite.

INTRODUCTION

Percutaneous thermal ablation techniques offer a minimally invasive alternative to surgery in which a needle probe is placed into a tumor and the offending tissue is killed by heating or cooling under image guidance. Typically, the tumor and a surrounding cuff of normal tissue, the ablation margin, are ablated. The usefulness and indications for these procedures have steadily increased as data demonstrating the safety and efficacy of ablation have grown.[1,2] Anesthesiologists are essential in effective periprocedural and procedural management. In this article, we describe common ablation techniques, image guidance modalities, and implications for anesthesiologists.

Disclosure Statement: No Disclosures.
[a] Department of Radiology, Brigham and Women's Hospital, Harvard Medical School, 75 Francis Street, Boston, MA 02115, USA; [b] Department of Anesthesiology, Vanderbilt University Medical Center, 1301 Medical Center Drive, 4648 TVC, Nashville, TN 37232, USA
* Corresponding author.
E-mail address: jason.lane@vanderbilt.edu

Anesthesiology Clin 35 (2017) 617–626
http://dx.doi.org/10.1016/j.anclin.2017.07.007

ABLATION TECHNIQUES

The most common percutaneous thermal ablation modalities currently used are radiofrequency ablation (RFA), microwave ablation (MWA), and cryoablation (CA).

Radiofrequency Ablation

RFA is a heat-based thermal ablation modality.[3] The RFA probe applies an electric current that travels through the patient to a grounding pad placed elsewhere on the patient's body (typically on the abdominal wall or leg, away from the procedural site). The current concentrates at the needle tip, resulting in localized heating at this location. When the tissue reaches temperatures exceeding 50°C, tissue coagulative necrosis occurs.[3] The duration of an ablation procedure depends on the number and size of tumors to be ablated, difficulty of the probe placement, and image guidance modality. Procedures generally last between 1 and 3 hours.

RFA is most commonly performed under ultrasound or computed tomography (CT) guidance. Although the ablation margin is not usually well-visualized with these modalities, image guidance remains essential to ensure accurate needle placement and to limit complications. Additionally, indirect signs of tumor ablation, such as formation of gas bubbles or subtle tissue attenuation changes, may be used to estimate the ablation zone. Recent advances in contrast-enhanced ultrasound imaging also have shown the ability to depict the ablation zone.[4] MRI is used less frequently because it is more expensive and time consuming, but it may be useful in ablation of tumors that are otherwise not visible by CT or ultrasound imaging. MRI often provides greater anatomic detail of adjacent structures, and therefore may be preferred for ablation close to critical structures. PET/CT guidance is also less common, but is increasing in usefulness and will likely play a greater role given its potential for immediate evaluation of the ablation margin and residual tumor.[5]

Microwave Ablation

MWA also involves the placement of a needle probe into the tumor under image guidance. The probe acts as an antenna that transmits microwave energy into the surrounding tissue; this energy results in rapid molecular realignments (dielectric hysteresis), which cause rapid tissue heating and destruction.[6,7] Unlike RFA, no grounding pad is required to be placed on the patient's body surface. MWA typically creates a more uniform ablation zone with more rapid heating relative to RFA, partly because the microwaves are capable of passing through charred and necrotic tissues more effectively. MWA has also demonstrated better clinical outcomes in the treatment of larger tumors (>5 cm) compared with RFA.[8]

MWA is also most commonly performed under ultrasound or CT guidance owing to relative ease of use and lower cost. MR and PET/CT guidance are being used with increasing frequency for the same reasons discussed for RF ablation guidance.

Cryoablation

CA relies on rapid cooling of tissue to kill tumors.[9,10] Cooling is achieved by rapid expansion of a gas (eg, argon) within the needle probe, with temperatures of at least −40°C resulting in effective ablation. After cooling, tissue is thawed for several minutes. Cycles of freezing and thawing result in cell death by multiple mechanisms, including direct immediate cellular toxicity, delayed apoptosis, and ischemic damage.[9] Each freezing and thawing cycle is repeated at least twice with each cycle lasting 5 to 20 minutes. CA typically takes longer than RFA and MWA owing to the requirement for multiple freeze–thaw cycles and use of multiple probes.

Unlike microwave and RF ablation, the CA zone is clearly visualized using CT, MR, or ultrasound guidance (although the deep ablation margin is not well seen with ultrasound imaging owing to shadowing by ice). Therefore, CA is often preferred for tumors close to critical structures that can be damaged inadvertently during the ablation and for smaller tumors in which the duration of the procedure is comparable with MW and RF ablation. In instances where larger tumors are ablated, multiple probes are placed 1 to 2 cm apart and within 1 cm of the outer tumor edge to ensure complete coverage.

Postprocedural Management and Potential Complications

Immediately after the ablation procedure, a sterile cover is placed at the skin entry site. Postprocedural imaging of the area of interest is performed to document postablation changes and assess for immediate complications. Outpatients are either discharged the same day or admitted for observation, laboratory follow-up, and possible additional imaging. These patients are initially placed at bed rest for at least 3 hours with a gradual increase in activity and diet as tolerated.

During the observation period, the patient is monitored for immediate complications, including bleeding, pneumothorax, damage to adjacent structures (eg, ureter after renal ablations, gallbladder or bowel after liver ablations), or electrolyte abnormalities.[10] Patients may also develop postablation syndrome after treatment of large tumors characterized by flulike symptoms. Postablation syndrome symptoms are typically treated conservatively, and resolve within 1 to 2 weeks after the ablation. An extensive ablation may result in myoglobinemia and myoglobinuria with subsequent acute renal failure. These complications treated with hydration and/or urine alkalinization with sodium bicarbonate.[11,12] Cases of severe thrombocytopenia requiring platelet transfusions have been reported after extensive liver CA.[13] A systemic response to tissue necrosis may rarely result in a "cryoshock" phenomenon that can result in multiorgan failure.

IMAGING GUIDANCE MODALITIES
Computed Tomography

CT has been an essential diagnostic tool since its development in the early 1970s. Since then, advances in spiral and multidetector CT techniques as well as increased computational power have allowed more rapid and higher quality image acquisition that has paved the way for CT-guided interventions, including ablation. CT fluoroscopy was developed in the 1990s and represented another major advancement in image-guided intervention. CT fluoroscopy has allowed real-time imaging by interventional radiology in the procedure room.[14] Large-bore CT scanners and portable scanners with arms that rotate around the patient are also available for claustrophobic or large patients.

Most CT interventional suites allow both diagnostic CT and CT fluoroscopy to be performed during the procedure. Diagnostic spiral CT allows high-resolution images to be taken in a region of interest and is commonly used for initial procedure planning, needle confirmation before biopsy or ablation, troubleshooting, and postprocedural evaluation of the initial postablation appearance and any potential complications. Diagnostic spiral CT scanning has higher radiation doses and therefore personnel must briefly leave the room during image acquisition. CT fluoroscopy is used most commonly to track small needle adjustments during the procedure in real time or near real time. Flouroscopy is controlled with a foot pedal and/or control pad placed at the side of the CT table. Although the resolution of CT fluoroscopy is relatively low, this is often sufficient for needle localization, allowing the interventional radiologist and other staff to remain in the room with the patient. CT fluoroscopy is associated with lower radiation, and can significantly reduce procedure times.

Radiation doses are reported as CT dose index and dose–length product, which are measured in grays and gray-centimeters, respectively. Exceeding recommended radiation doses can lead to immediate adverse effects (most commonly radiation skin burns) and also increases the patient's cumulative risk of cancer and organ damage.[15] Therefore, it is important to minimize radiation exposure to the patient. This concept is often referred to as the ALARA principle (as low as reasonably achievable).[16,17] To achieve ALARA, prior imaging is carefully reviewed so the planning CT scan can be limited only to the area of interest. In addition, lead drapes cover areas of the patient outside of region of interest, intermittent (pulsed) fluoroscopy is used instead of continuous imaging, and only a few images showing the needle tip and surrounding structures are obtained during CT fluoroscopy imaging.

The largest source of radiation to personnel in the CT suite is scattered radiation from the patient's body.[15] Direct radiation from the scan beam and source leakage also contribute to unintended personnel exposure. Radiation levels diminish exponentially with distance; therefore, even small incremental increases in distance from the patient and scanner significantly reduce personnel doses.

PET-Computed Tomography

Positron emission tomography (PET) is commonly used for cancer detection and staging. The most common radiotracer used in cancer PET imaging is F-18 fluorodeoxyglucose (FDG), which is a glucose analog that is taken up by metabolically active tissues such as tumors. The patient fasts for 4 to 6 hours before tracer injection with the goal of reducing glucose levels below 150 mg/dL; since glucose competes with FDG for cellular uptake, this maximizes tumor FDG uptake and visualization. PET images are taken approximately 60 minutes after injection, and are combined with low resolution CT, which allows better localization and evaluation of anatomic detail. Each "slice" takes approximately 1 to 5 minutes to acquire.

PET-CT has gained significant recent interest in guiding ablation procedures as it has the ability to visualize residual tumor and ensure complete tumor ablation, which is not always possible with CT, ultrasound, or MR.[5,18] In addition to slow image acquisition time, the main limitation of PET-CT is misalignment of the PET and CT images, which occurs if there is change in patient position between CT and PET image acquisition. This misalignment occurs most commonly owing to breathing, and is therefore especially problematic for lesions near the diaphragm. In these cases, respiratory triggered acquisitions, careful sedation/ventilation to minimize diaphragmatic excursion during breathing, and special breath-hold techniques (particularly under general anesthesia) can be useful to reduce mis-registration.[5]

Ultrasound Imaging

Ultrasound is a very versatile and relatively inexpensive imaging modality commonly used for interventional guidance of many procedures, including ablations. Ultrasound signal detection relies on the transmission of acoustic waves into tissue and measurement of the reflected acoustic signal by a handheld probe. Advantages of ultrasound include real-time image guidance and ability to easily change the imaging plane as needed to localize the needle and adjacent tissues. In addition, there is no ionizing radiation and there are no significant risks to the patient at energies used for standard diagnostic ultrasound applications and ablation guidance. Doppler ultrasound allows evaluation of vessels and the recent development and FDA approval of ultrasound contrast agents allows for evaluation of tissue vascularity. Ultrasound contrast agents have been shown to be safe, with reported life-threatening anaphylaxis rates of 0.001%,[19] and can be useful to assess for complete tumor ablation.[4]

Limitations of US are the inability to penetrate bone or air, which precludes visualization of lung parenchyma and structures in the abdomen that are deep to bowel. Ultrasound also has limited penetration depths, which can be problematic in larger patients or in evaluation of deep anatomic structures.

MRI

MRI uses timed magnetic gradients and radiofrequency pulses to image tissues. Advantages of MRI are its high intrinsic spatial resolution and ability to image in any anatomic plane. In addition, MRI can often visualize tumors that are not well seen by other modalities. The use of diffusion weighted sequences can be useful to target cellular tumor,[20] and temperature sensitive sequences can be used to assess thermal effects during ablation.[21,22]

MRI is less commonly used compared to ultrasound and CT owing to its high cost and relatively slow imaging and procedural time. In addition, the long acquisition times can result in significant motion artifact from breathing and shifting of patient position. However, MRI technology continues to develop with shorter scan times and increased signal to noise ratio, making it a more practical ablation guidance modality.[23,24]

Although both open and closed bore MRI systems have been used during interventions, closed bore systems have remained more popular owing to the development of systems with larger gantries and higher field strengths. Wide (70 cm or larger) and short (125–150 cm) bore high-field systems have been developed and increase access to the patient during interventions. These new scanners also allow the interventional radiologist to minimize the number of times that the patient is moved into and out of the scanner.

Open MRI systems are also available and can be useful in patients that are large or claustrophobic. These systems allow more flexibility and greater access to the patient during the procedure; however, they are usually of significantly lower field strength (0.2–1.0 T), resulting in lower spatial resolution and signal strength. In addition, open systems have longer image acquisition times, requiring longer breath holds.

IMPLICATIONS FOR ANESTHESIA

In this section, we discuss unique challenges for the anesthesiologist in navigating the interventional suite and providing effective aesthesia during image guided percutaneous ablation.

Positioning in the Interventional Suite

Patient, personnel, and equipment positioning can be particularly challenging in the interventional suite given the spatial constraints imposed by the imaging equipment (particularly for CT, PET-CT, and MRI). Depending on the location of the tumor and optimal interventional approach, the patient may be placed in prone, supine, or oblique position on the table. Before preparation of the sterile field, the patient should be positioned such that he/she is comfortable, the anesthesiologist must have easy access to all lines, tubes, and monitoring devices, and the interventional radiologist has access to the imaging controls, ablation tools, and patient needle entry site.

The interventional radiologist is typically positioned on one side of the gantry toward the feet of the patient, while the anesthesiologist is positioned on the opposite side near the patient's head. The patient is moved into and out of the scanner gantry during the procedure; therefore, necessary lines and monitoring equipment should have enough length to allow free and uninhibited patient translation. In addition, while the scanner bed is moved, all personnel should be vigilant to ensure that these lines and tubes are not inadvertently pulled, removed, or damaged.

Patient Monitoring

Patient monitoring can also be challenging, particularly with CT, PET-CT, and MRI guidance. During fluoroscopic CT and MRI image acquisition, personnel may stay in the interventional suite as long as they have appropriate protective equipment (eg, lead apron for CT fluoroscopy and ear plugs for MRI). During diagnostic spiral CT acquisition, staff should step out of the imaging room and into an adjacent control room owing to the higher radiation doses. A video camera and microphone is usually available to allow constant visual and auditory monitoring. Patient vital signs are also typically projected on a monitor in the control room; if not, the monitoring console should be positioned such that it can be seen from outside the imaging suite.

MRI provides additional challenges to patient care and monitoring. Continuous ECG monitoring is important during ablation. MRI compatible 3- and 4- lead ECG devices have lower signal strength and are not sensitive for detection of silent cardiac ischemia; MRI conditional 12-lead ECG has recently been developed but has not been extensively clinically tested or validated.[25] Therefore, patients at high risk for active ischemic heart disease should not have ablation procedures performed under MRI guidance.

In addition, patient monitoring equipment in the interventional MRI suite must be MRI compatible (eg, will not harm the patient, will not affect image quality, and will function as intended in the presence of a strong magnetic field). Standard anesthesia equipment is often MRI incompatible or MRI conditional (only appropriate under certain field strengths and conditions); therefore, extreme care should be taken and appropriate documentation should be thoroughly reviewed before bringing equipment into the MRI scan room. The anesthesia literature has multiple examples of injuries that have occurred to patients in MRI scanner under sedation or general anesthesia when a ferro-magnetic piece of equipment is brought into Zone 4 of the MRI scanner. The results are often disastrous at best, and fatal at worst. Quenching (shut-down) of the MRI magnet is also typically required to remove the metallic object from the MRI magnet. In the case of a hospital gurney or oxygen cylinder brought into Zone 4, extrication of the patient is typically dependent upon rapid MRI magnet quenching. Resultant energy from the magnet must be released, typically into a container of liquid helium atop the MRI magenet, which rapidly evaporates, and is vented outside the building as gaseous helium. When inappropriate venting of gaseous helium occurs, and it vents into the MRI scanner room, the results can be life-threatening for all involved. An immediate hypoxic environment is created in the scanner room. It can be difficult to get access to the patient owing to gas pressure differences in the scanner room compared to outside (Zone 3). Use of an MRI pressure equalization kit is often required to gain access to the patient. While rare events indeed, knowledge about these potential dangers is important for the radiology and anesthesiology teams to ensure patient safety while in the MRI scanner.

Sedation and Pain Management

At our institution, a thorough outpatient pre-procedural assessment is performed by an anesthesiologist 1 week before the procedure, and ablation is usually performed under monitored anesthesia care (MAC). Conscious sedation is sufficient for most patients, but general anesthesia is occasionally required in patients whose history prevents sufficient pain control or comfortable positioning (eg, history of prior high dose narcotics, anterior abdominal wounds in patients who must lie prone, tolerance to benzodiazepines, etc...).

The ability to have reproducible breathing and diaphragmatic excursion is important for targeting and ablation of tumors close to the diaphragm, such as those in the liver. It is often useful to begin sedation before initial imaging so that sedation-related breathing changes are incorporated into pre-procedural planning and positioning. During the procedure, reproducible breath holds allow safe needle advancement at the same point of the patient's respiratory cycle (most often end expiration). For conscious sedation patients, using lighter sedation during needle advancement allows patient cooperation with breath holding. For general anesthesia patients, interruption of ventilation at a consistent level serves the same purpose.

Although ablation is generally well tolerated, there are specific times during the procedure during which the patient may experience an increased level of discomfort. There is often increased discomfort at the time of initial local anesthesia administration and needle placement, puncture of sensitive structures such as the peritoneum or hepatic capsule, and during active tissue heating or freezing. CA is associated with less pain compared to RFA or MWA, but typically patients receive more sedation and analgesia during the active ablation regardless of modality.

Ablation of tumors adjacent to sensitive structures may lead to increased postprocedural pain. Peri-diaphragmatic ablation can lead to referred shoulder pain that can remain for days or even weeks after the procedure. In addition, artificial ascites or pneumoperitoneum is occasionally introduced during the procedure to protect adjacent structures; if air and/or fluid is not sufficiently drained after the procedure, this may also result in abdominal or referred shoulder pain.[26] Therefore, awareness of the procedural details, location, and extent of the ablation is important in postprocedural pain management and patient counseling.

Personnel Safety

As discussed previously, all staff in the interventional suite are exposed to radiation during CT fluoroscopy; owing to cumulative effects of radiation, it is important for everyone, and particularly those who participate in a large number of such interventions, to minimize exposure. Whenever possible, personnel should stand away from scanner and ensure that no part of their body extends into the beam. In addition, those in the room during CT fluoroscopy must wear a lead apron with a 0.35 mm lead equivalent and a thyroid shield. Protective lead goggles are not required but can reduce the risk of cataracts.[27,28]

There is potential for radiation exposure to personnel during PET imaging from positron-emitting radiotracers, and therefore personnel should maintain distance from the patient when possible.[29] Lead aprons used for CT do not stop the high photon energies of PET radiopharmaceuticals and are therefore not typically used.

MRI does not utilize ionizing radiation, but has its own set of unique safety considerations for personnel.[30,31] Metallic ferromagnetic objects brought into the room may become projectiles with potential for patient or staff injury and damage to equipment. Anyone with implanted devices or foreign metal objects in their body should have thorough screening before entering the interventional suite. Finally, coils used in MRI imaging create high decibel noise that can result in temporary or even permanent hearing loss, and therefore ear plugs are recommended for everyone in the room.

Ablation of Adrenal Masses

Ablation of adrenal tumors has been shown to be effective, but this procedure may result in life-threatening catecholamine-induced hypertensive crisis.[32] This complication may occur with ablation of any adrenal tumor, but most likely it will occur when residual adrenal tissue is present.[33] During CA, catecholamine-associated hypertensive crisis is most common during the thaw phase of the freeze-thaw cycle, while it is seen during the heating phase of MWA and RFA. Hypertensive crisis can also occur immediately after the procedure.

Pretreatment with alpha-blockade has been shown to reduce the risk and severity of hypertensive crisis and is recommended before all adrenal ablations.[32] However, this is not preventative, and both the interventional radiologist and anesthesia team should be prepared to manage catecholamine-induced crisis during or immediately after the procedure.

SUMMARY

Image guided percutaneous ablation is increasingly common in clinical practice and the anesthesiologist and interventional radiologist must work together to ensure a safe and effective outcome. The anesthesia team must be aware of common ablation techniques, complications, and image guidance modalities reviewed here in order to adapt to the unique challenges associated with the interventional suite.

REFERENCES

1. Hoffmann R, Rempp H, Keßler D-E, et al. MR-guided microwave ablation in hepatic tumours: initial results in clinical routine. Eur Radiol 2017;27(4):1467–76. Available at: http://link.springer.com/10.1007/s00330-016-4517-x. Accessed November 19, 2016.

2. Yu J, Liang P, Yu X-L, et al. Us-guided percutaneous microwave ablation versus open radical nephrectomy for small renal cell carcinoma: intermediate-term results. Radiology 2014;270(3):880–7.

3. Hong K, Georgiades C. Radiofrequency ablation: mechanism of action and devices. J Vasc Interv Radiol 2010;21(8 Suppl):S179–86.

4. Lu M, Yu X, Li A, et al. Comparison of contrast enhanced ultrasound and contrast enhanced CT or MRI in monitoring percutaneous thermal ablation procedure in patients with hepatocellular carcinoma: a Multi-Center Study in China. Ultrasound Med Biol 2007;33(11):1736–49.

5. Shyn PB, Tatli S, Sahni VA, et al. PET/CT-guided percutaneous liver mass biopsies and ablations: targeting accuracy of a single 20 s breath-hold PET acquisition. Clin Radiol 2014;69(4):410–5.

6. Lubner MG, Brace CL, Hinshaw JL, et al. Microwave tumor ablation: mechanism of action, clinical results, and devices. J Vasc Interv Radiol 2010;21(Suppl 8): S192–203. Available at: http://dx.doi.org/10.1016/j.jvir.2010.04.007.

7. Simon CJ, Dupuy DE, Mayo-Smith WW. Microwave ablation: principles and applications. Radiographics 2005;25(Suppl 1):S69–83. Available at: http://pubs.rsna.org/doi/abs/10.1148/rg.25si055501. Accessed April 23, 2016.

8. Thamtorawat S, Hicks RM, Yu J, et al. Preliminary outcome of microwave ablation of hepatocellular carcinoma: breaking the 3-cm barrier? J Vasc Interv Radiol 2016;27(5):623–30.

9. Erinjeri JP, Clark TWI. Cryoablation: mechanism of action and devices. J Vasc Interv Radiol 2010;21(8):S187–91.

10. Bhagavatula S, Shyn PB. Image-guided renal interventions. Radiol Clin North Am 2017;55(2):359–71.

11. Silverman SG, Tuncali K, Adams DF, et al. MR imaging-guided percutaneous cryotherapy of liver tumors: initial experience. Radiology 2000;217(3):657–64. Available at: http://www.ncbi.nlm.nih.gov/pubmed/11110925.

12. Foltz G. Image-guided percutaneous ablation of hepatic malignancies. Semin Intervent Radiol 2014;31(2):180–6. Available at: http://www.ncbi.nlm.nih.gov/pubmed/25071304. Accessed November 19, 2016.

13. Tatli S, Morrison PR, Tuncali K, et al. Interventional MRI for Oncologic Applications. Tech Vasc Interv Radiol 2007;10(2):159–70.

14. Begemann PGC. Ct-guided interventions: indications, technique, and pitfalls. In: Mahnken AH, Ricke J, editors. CT-and MR-Guided Interventions in Radiology. Berlin, Heidelberg: Springer; 2013. p. 11–24.

15. Kloeckner R, Dos Santos DP, Schneider J, et al. Radiation exposure in CT-guided interventions. Eur J Radiol 2013;82(12):2253–7.

16. Sarti M, Brehmer WP, Gay SB. Low-dose techniques in CT-guided interventions. RadioGraphics 2012;32(4):1109–19. Available at: http://www.ncbi.nlm.nih.gov/pubmed/22786997. Accessed December 1, 2016.

17. Jungnickel K. Radiation protection during CT-guided interventions. In: Mahnken AH, Ricke J, editors. CT- and MR-guided interventions in radiology. New York: Springer New York; 2009. p. 35–8.

18. Ryan ER, Sofocleous CT, Schöder H, et al. Split-dose technique for FDG PET/CT-guided percutaneous ablation: a method to facilitate lesion targeting and to provide immediate assessment of treatment effectiveness. Radiology 2013;268(1):288–95. Available at: http://pubs.rsna.org/doi/10.1148/radiol.13121462. Accessed December 1, 2016.

19. Claudon M, Dietrich C, Choi B, et al. Guidelines and good clinical practice recommendations for contrast enhanced ultrasound (CEUS) in the liver – Update 2012. Ultraschall Med 2012;34(01):11–29. Available at: http://www.thieme-connect.de/DOI/DOI?10.1055/s-0032-1325499. Accessed November 23, 2016.

20. Guimaraes MD, Gross JL, Chojniak R, et al. MRI-guided biopsy: a valuable procedure alternative to avoid the risks of ionizing radiation from diagnostic imaging methods. Cardiovasc Intervent Radiol 2014;37(3):858–60. Available at: http://link.springer.com/10.1007/s00270-013-0677-0. Accessed November 13, 2016.

21. Jolesz FA. From biopsy to intraoperative imaging: MRI-guided procedures. In: Jolesz F, Young I, editors. Interventional MR, techniques and clinical experience. London: Martin Dunitz Ltd; 1998. p. 1–8.

22. Tempany CMC, Stewart EA, McDannold N, et al. MR imaging–guided focused ultrasound surgery of uterine leiomyomas: a feasibility study. Radiology 2003;226(3):897–905. Available at: http://pubs.rsna.org/doi/10.1148/radiol.2271020395. Accessed December 2, 2016.

23. Edelstein W, Bottomley P, Hart H. Signal, noise, and contrast in nuclear magnetic resonance (NMR) imaging. J Comput Assist Tomogr 1983;7(3):391–401. Available at: http://www.jcat.org/pt/re/jcat/abstract.00004728-198306000-00001.htm.

24. Hoult DI, Lauterbur PC. The sensitivity of the zeugmatographic experiment involving human samples. J Magn Reson 1979;34(2):425–33.

25. Tse ZTH, Dumoulin CL, Clifford GD, et al. A 1.5T MRI-conditional 12-lead electrocardiogram for MRI and intra-MR intervention. Magn Reson Med 2014;71(3):1336–47. Available at: http://www.ncbi.nlm.nih.gov/pubmed/23580148. Accessed November 13, 2016.

26. Bhagavatula SK, Chick JFB, Chauhan NR, et al. Artificial ascites and pneumoperitoneum to facilitate thermal ablation of liver tumors: a pictorial essay. Abdom

Radiol (NY) 2017;42(2):620–30. Available at: http://www.ncbi.nlm.nih.gov/pubmed/27665483. Accessed December 1, 2016.

27. Anastasian ZH, Strozyk D, Meyers PM, et al. Radiation exposure of the anesthesiologist in the neurointerventional suite. Anesthesiology 2011;114(3):512–20. Available at: http://anesthesiology.pubs.asahq.org/Article.aspx?doi=10.1097/ALN.0b013e31820c2b81. Accessed October 14, 2016.

28. Rubin D. Anesthesia for ambulatory diagnostic and therapeutic radiology procedures. Anesthesiol Clin 2014;32(2):371–80.

29. Povoski SP, Sarikaya I, White WC, et al. Comprehensive evaluation of occupational radiation exposure to intraoperative and perioperative personnel from 18F-FDG radioguided surgical procedures. Eur J Nucl Med Mol Imaging 2008; 35(11):2026–34. Available at: http://www.ncbi.nlm.nih.gov/pubmed/18618106. Accessed February 19, 2017.

30. Kraff O, Ladd ME. MR safety update 2015: where do the risks come from;? Curr Radiol Rep 2016;4(6):1–6.

31. Kanal E, Barkovich AJ, Bell C, et al. ACR guidance document on MR safe practices: 2013. J Magn Reson Imaging 2013;37(3):501–30.

32. Welch BT, Atwell TD, Nichols DA, et al. Percutaneous image-guided adrenal cryoablation: procedural considerations and technical success. Radiology 2011; 258(1):301–7.

33. Schenker MP, Martin R, Shyn PB, et al. Interventional radiology and anesthesia. Anesthesiol Clin 2009;27(1):87–94.

Catheterization Laboratory

Structural Heart Disease, Devices, and Transcatheter Aortic Valve Replacement

Paul N. Fiorilli, MD[a], Saif Anwaruddin, MD[b], Elizabeth Zhou, MD[c], Ronak Shah, MD[c],*

KEYWORDS

- TVAR • Left atrial occlusion device • Cardiac catheterization laboratory
- Endovascular edge to edge mitral valve repair

KEY POINTS

- Transcatheter aortic valve replacement is approved for those patients considered intermediate risk for open heart surgery and is performed under monitored anesthesia care or sedation.
- TAVR is a high-risk procedure, and the team must be prepared for immediate cardiopulmonary bypass and resuscitation.
- Endovascular edge-to-edge mitral valve repair is approved for patients who are high risk for open mitral valve repair. It is like an open Alfieri stitch repair, increasing coaptation between the anterior and posterior leaflets.
- A left atrial occlusion device is an alternative to chronic anticoagulation therapy. Deployment is done under general anesthesia with transesophageal echocardiography guidance.

INTRODUCTION

Medicine is rapidly evolving. The advent of newer technologies allow for the same outcome with less invasive surgery, shorter duration of hospital stay, and faster recovery times. The cardiac catheterization laboratory (CCL) is at the forefront of

Disclosure Statement: The authors have nothing to disclose.

[a] Interventional Cardiology, Cardiovascular Division, Department of Anesthesiology and Critical Care, Hospital of the University of Pennsylvania, 3400 Spruce Street, Philadelphia, PA 19104, USA; [b] Transcatheter Valve Program, Department of Anesthesiology and Critical Care, Perelman School of Medicine at the University of Pennsylvania, Hospital of the University of Pennsylvania, 3400 Spruce Street, Philadelphia, PA 19104, USA; [c] Adult Cardiothoracic Anesthesiology, Department of Anesthesiology and Critical Care, Hospital of the University of Pennsylvania, 3400 Spruce Street, Philadelphia, PA 19104, USA
* Corresponding author.
E-mail address: Ronak.Shah@uphs.upenn.edu

Anesthesiology Clin 35 (2017) 627–639
http://dx.doi.org/10.1016/j.anclin.2017.07.008
1932-2275/17/© 2017 Elsevier Inc. All rights reserved.

implementing minimally invasive procedures, such as catheter-based therapies. The CCL advanced coronary artery disease treatment, with the ability to correct ischemia-causing disease without requiring open heart surgery. Many procedures performed in the CCL are done so without the assistance of an anesthesiologist. These procedures include diagnostic catheterizations, percutaneous coronary interventions, and balloon mitral valvuloplasty. These patients receive a generous amount of local anesthetic and intravenous sedation for their procedures. The sedation is routinely administered by certified nurses under the direction of the interventionalist. Although most patients in the CCL are managed without an anesthesiologist, some procedures do require general anesthesia or more complicated sedation for the procedure. The anesthetic approach to procedures such as transcatheter aortic valve replacement (TAVR), left atrial appendage closure and mitral clip repair varies from center to center.

Because most cases done in the CCL are performed without an anesthesiologist, these laboratories are not typically part of the main operating area, but rather on a separate cardiology floor. When requested, anesthesiologists must be prepared to handle potentially critically ill patients in an unfamiliar non–operating room setting. Non–operating room suites may lack readily available resources traditionally found in the operating theater, such as additional anesthesia support and familiar operating room equipment.

AORTIC STENOSIS

One of the biggest advances in the CCL is in the treatment of aortic stenosis. Patients typically present with aortic stenosis in their sixth decade of life, and if severe enough will warrant surgical replacement or a surgical aortic valve replacement (SAVR). Aortic valve replacement is the most common valvular surgery performed. Unfortunately, not every patient is eligible for a SAVR procedure owing to increased risk because of multiple comorbidities. Patients not eligible for SAVR are managed medically.

INTRODUCTION TO TRANSCATHETER AORTIC VALVE REPLACEMENT

TAVR was first approved by the US Food and Drug Administration (FDA) in November of 2011. In that time, TAVR has emerged as an effective treatment alternative to traditional SAVR in patients with severe aortic stenosis who are at intermediate risk or high risk for morbidity and mortality with traditional surgery.[1,2] The benefit of TAVR in patients who are deemed inoperable for surgery has also been established.[3] Currently, the American Heart Association/American College of Cardiology 2017 valvular guidelines focused update recommends TAVR for patients who are at prohibitive risk for SAVR (class 1, level of evidence A).[4] In addition, TAVR is considered equivalent to SAVR in patients with aortic stenosis who have high surgical risk for SAVR (class 1, level of evidence A).[4] Last, TAVR is considered a reasonable alternative to SAVR in patients with aortic stenosis who have an intermediate surgical risk for SAVR (class IIA, level of evidence B).[4] As indications for TAVR have expanded, the number of TAVR procedures performed has steadily increased. From 2012 to 2015, the volume of TAVR in the United States has increased from 4627 procedures in 2012 to 24,808 procedures in 2015.[5] Over that same period, in-hospital mortality from TAVR decreased from 5.9% to 2.9%.[5] Overall, TAVR has become much more prevalent, and the procedural outcomes have continued to improve.

TRANSCATHETER AORTIC VALVE REPLACEMENT VERSUS MEDICAL THERAPY

In patients who are considered prohibitive risk for surgery for aortic stenosis, medical therapy has long been the mainstay of treatment. The use of TAVR in this patient population as compared with standard medical therapy was evaluated in the PARTNER B trial (using the Edwards SAPIEN system). In this trial, 358 patients underwent randomization to TAVR or medical therapy. The rate of death at 1 year was 30.7% in the TAVR group and 50.7% in the medical therapy group (hazard ratio of 0.55 with TAVR; $P<.001$).[3] The composite endpoint of death from any cause or repeat hospitalization was 42.5% in the TAVR group and 71.6% in the medical therapy group (hazard ratio of 0.46; $P<.001$).[3] These results were sustained at the 2-year follow-up.[6] Overall, in patients with severe aortic stenosis who are not considered operative candidates, TAVR has been shown to reduce mortality.

TRANSCATHETER AORTIC VALVE REPLACEMENT VERSUS SURGICAL THERAPY

Concomitantly, TAVR was compared with SAVR for patients considered high risk for SAVR. In the PARTNER A trial, 699 patients considered high risk for surgery were randomized to traditional SAVR or to TAVR (with a balloon-expandable valve delivered via the transfemoral [TF] or transaortic approach).[1] The rates of death from any cause were not statistically significant between the groups at 30 days (3.4% with TAVR vs 6.5% with SAVR; $P = .07$) or 1 year (24.2% with TAVR vs 26.8% with SAVR; $P = .44$). The rates of major stroke were higher in the TAVR group at both 30 days and 1 year, and vascular complications were higher in the TAVR group as well. The SAVR group experienced more frequent major bleeding and new-onset atrial fibrillation. Overall, in high-risk patients with severe aortic stenosis, TAVR and SAVR had similar rates of mortality with some differences in procedural risk.

Next, TAVR was compared with SAVR in patients with intermediate surgical risk. In the PARTNER 2 trial, 2032 patients were randomized to TAVR or SAVR.[2] The rate of death from any cause or disabling stroke was similar between the 2 groups. Interestingly, in the TF access cohort, TAVR resulted in a lower rate of death or disabling stroke as compared with SAVR (hazard ratio, 0.79; $P = .05$). Patients treated with TAVR had a lower incidence of acute renal failure, major bleeding, and new-onset atrial fibrillation. Alternatively, SAVR patients had a lower rate of major vascular complications and paravalvular regurgitation. Overall, these results suggest that TAVR is like SAVR in intermediate-risk patients with severe aortic stenosis undergoing aortic valve replacement. Notably, patients who have anatomy amenable to a TF approach may have improved outcomes compared with the traditional surgical approach.

The PARTNER trials involved the use of the Edwards SAPIEN balloon-expandable system. The Medtronic CoreValve Revalving system was evaluated in the US CoreValve Trial. In this trial, 795 patients who were deemed at high surgical risk were randomized to TAVR or SAVR. The TAVR group had a lower mortality (14.2% vs 19.1%; $P = .04$) at 1 year.[7] This led to the approval, in the United States, for the CoreValve System to treat high and prohibitive surgical risk patients. The intermediate-risk Medtronic trial, SURTAVI, was recently published. In this study, the rates of mortality between TAVR and SAVR were similar and met significance for noninferiority.[8]

ROUTES OF DELIVERY

There are several different methods of vascular access for valve delivery: TF, transapical, direct aortic, and transsubclavian (or transaxillary). Novel approaches, such as transcarotid and transcaval, have also been described. The TF approach is the most common approach worldwide and can be performed fully percutaneously using a "preclosure" technique.[9] The rates of vascular complications related to TF access have improved as the profiles of the delivery systems have decreased with the newer valve generations. The TF approach is the least invasive vascular approach. There are advantages and disadvantages of the other vascular access approaches, but all are more involved and more invasive then the TF approach and, consequently, TF access is considered the standard of care if the patient's anatomy is amenable.

TYPES OF TRANSCATHETER AORTIC VALVE REPLACEMENT VALVES

Currently, there are 2 types of valves that are approved in the United States by the FDA. This included the Edwards SAPIEN system (Edwards Lifesciences Corporation; Irvine, CA), and the Medtronic CoreValve Revalving system (Medtronic, Inc.; Minnesota, MN).

Edwards SAPIEN System

There are 2 Edwards SAPIEN aortic valves that approved for commercial use: the SAPIEN XT valve and the SAPIEN 3 valve. The SAPIEN valves are equine pericardial valves with a stainless steel framework that are balloon expandable. Notably, the SAPIEN XT valve is currently approved by the FDA for aortic valve-in-valve procedures. The SAPIEN 3 valve, the newest generation of the SAPIEN system, has a smaller device profile (smaller arterial sheath size) and a polyethylene terephthalate skirt. These 2 features have helped to improve vascular access site complications and to decrease incidence of paravalvular regurgitation after valve deployment. Significant paravalvular regurgitation after device deployment has been shown to correlate with worse short- and long-term mortality.[10–12]

Medtronic CoreValve Revalving System

The Medtronic CoreValve Revalving system differs from SAPIEN in that it has a self-expanding nitinol frame and is a porcine pericardial bioprosthesis. The Evolut R valve, the newest generation, is approved for valve-in-valve replacement, and is unique in that it is the only approved transcatheter valve that is recapturable.

COMPARISON OF TRANSCATHETER AORTIC VALVE REPLACEMENT VERSUS SURGICAL AORTIC VALVE REPLACEMENT

Several important periprocedural differences between TAVR and SAVR have emerged as the field of TAVR has developed. TAVR is a less invasive procedure than SAVR. Patients undergoing TAVR have been shown to have lower rates of acute renal failure, atrial fibrillation, major bleeding, and infection.[1,2] Importantly, the use of TAVR avoids the need for cardiopulmonary bypass. As discussed, patients who have TF access for TAVR have lower rates of death and disabling stroke as compared with SAVR.[2] In addition to these important periprocedural differences, TAVR also has notable hemodynamic advantages as well. As compared with SAVR, TAVR leads to a larger effective orifice area of the implanted valve.[13] This has been shown to lead to a lower incidence of patient–prosthesis mismatch.[14]

FUTURE DIRECTIONS FOR TRANSCATHETER AORTIC VALVE REPLACEMENT

The rapid development of TAVR and the significant improvements in valve delivery technology have revolutionized the treatment of aortic stenosis. As stated, the 2017 American Heart Association/American College of Cardiology valvular guidelines have indications for TAVR in intermediate, high, and prohibitive risk patients. Currently, trials are underway with TAVR in low-risk patients. The PARTNER III study will randomize low-risk patients 65 years of age or older to TAVR or SAVR. The trial is designed as a noninferiority study with a 1-year composite endpoint of death, stroke, or rehospitalization. The Medtronic low-risk trial will also evaluate the self-expanding prosthesis in low-risk patients. This trial has a 2-year composite endpoint of all-cause mortality or disabling stroke. As these trials forge ahead into low-risk populations, the implications for expansion of the use of this technology are significant.

ANESTHESIA PREEVALUATION

A complete preprocedure evaluation should be done to develop an intraoperative management plan. Although TAVR is considered minimally invasive, it remains a high-risk procedure. In addition to the procedure itself predisposing the patient to increased risk, this patient population has been already deemed too high risk for open heart surgery. These patients often present to the CCL with comorbidities that will affect intraoperative management. Certain conditions such as low ejection fraction, right ventricular dysfunction, coronary artery disease, chronic obstructive pulmonary disease, coronary artery disease, pulmonary hypertension, or mitral regurgitation should be carefully evaluated with additional and appropriate studies to help better assess risk and severity.

1. A complete patient history detailing allergies, medications, and past medical and surgical history, including any adverse reactions with any anesthesia exposure.
2. Objective data must be reviewed to assess heart, liver, kidney, and pulmonary function to help guide the anesthesia management.
3. Assessment for obstructive sleep apnea and functional status of patient.

Initially, at our institution all TAVRs were performed under general anesthesia with continuous invasive arterial blood pressure monitoring, pulmonary artery catheter and a transesophageal echocardiography (TEE). Patients were sometimes extubated in the operating room depending on hemodynamic stability. Narcotic and paralysis are used sparingly to help facilitate extubation at the end. Our interventionalists have become more familiar with the device as well as the development of smaller delivery systems. Initially, a 22-Fr delivery system was used, which has been reduced to a 14-Fr system. This decrease in size has reduced vascular complications.[15] For these reasons, the combination of a local anesthetic and sedation has increased for the primary anesthetic.

Sedation may be further categorized as mild, moderate, or deep when administered by nonanesthesiologists.[16,17] Sedation delivered by an anesthesiologist is referred to as monitored anesthesia care (MAC).[18] Sedation for TF TAVR should be considered unless the patient is unable tolerate it, or if the center is a low-volume TAVR institution. However, transapical or transaortic TAVR should be done under general anesthesia because surgical access is required for valve deployment, although there are reported cases of regional anesthesia being used for these routes of delivery.[19-21]

Once a complete preoperative evaluation has been done, patients' tolerance for MAC anesthesia with local anesthetic is determined. At our institution, all patients undergoing a TF TAVR are initially considered for MAC. If patients cannot comfortably lay flat for an extended period, then the patient will receive general anesthesia with an endotracheal tube. Patients often present with chronic back pain that prohibits them from lying flat. Additionally, some patients with extensive pulmonary disease requiring supplemental oxygen therapy may not tolerate sedation. These patients might require an even higher fraction of inspired oxygen under MAC. Patients with intolerable dyspnea while lying flat will not endure MAC for an extended period. Intolerance to lying flat is an absolute contraindication for a MAC anesthetic at our institution. In the past, a reduced left ventricular or right ventricular function, or increased pulmonary artery pressures, was a contraindication to MAC. However, our increasing familiarity with the technique and an evolving device, recent data show MAC patients experienced fewer complications.[22]

Sedation or MAC provides several advantages over general anesthesia. General anesthesia increases peripheral vasodilation and suppresses myocardial function, which may ultimately lead to increased pharmacologic support to maintain hemodynamic stability. Sedation allows clinicians to continuously evaluate the patient's mental status throughout the TAVR procedure. TVAR does increase risk of neurologic injury.[23–26]

A large retrospective study in the United States reviewed more than 10,997 TF TAVR cases, in which 15.8% of patients received moderate sedation. The study found lower rates of 30-day mortality or stroke, and a shorter duration of hospital stay associated with the sedation group. This is one of the first studies indicating a mortality benefit for sedation.[22]

At our institution, MAC is accomplished using a combination of low-dose remifentanil and dexmedetomidine. During sheath placement, small boluses of etomidate may be administered to help the patient tolerate periods of discomfort without compromising hemodynamic stability or causing ventilatory depression.[27]

Although sedation should be considered the default anesthetic for TF TAVR procedures, patients who are unable tolerate MAC, or deemed a poor candidate for MAC, general anesthesia with an endotracheal tube should be used. In the United States, general anesthesia is the most perform anesthetic technique for these procedures. However, this percentage decreasing from 95.1% in 2012% to 83.1% in 2015, suggesting that interventionalists are becoming more comfortable in performing the procedure, leading to more sedation use for patients.[28]

Although sedation and MAC are increasing in popularity, general anesthesia also provides multiple benefits. Positive pressure ventilation with an endotracheal tube will help to minimize the risk of aspiration. Apnea can be provided during valve positioning and deployment to help reduce interference from respiratory movement. Finally, placement of TEE is better tolerated by patients who are under general anesthesia with an endotracheal tube.[29] Other than patient refusal, there are no contraindications to general anesthesia.

Induction of general anesthesia is a risky process that may result in death owing to hemodynamic instability in these very sick patients. Patients with critical aortic stenosis typically present with hypertrophic left ventricles that require a higher systemic pressure for adequate coronary perfusion. Preinduction continuous invasive arterial blood pressure monitoring and defibrillator pads should be included with the standard American Society of Anesthesiologists' (ASA) monitors. Etomidate or narcotic-based induction (ie, fentanyl) should be considered to minimize any significant myocardial depression or decreases in mean arterial pressures. General management for patients with aortic stenosis include avoiding tachycardia to allow the ventricles more filling time to ensure appropriate preload and avoiding hypotension to ensure coronary perfusion and maintain sinus rhythm. Patients in atrial fibrillation lose their atrial contraction. The LV receives less preload. Phenylephrine should be considered if pharmacologic intervention is required to increase systemic pressure because it will increase afterload and help to reduce the heart rate via reflexive bradycardia.[30]

MONITORING

In addition to standard ASA monitors, external defibrillating pads are applied. Regardless of the anesthetic technique, a peripheral large-bore intravenous line and a radial artery catheter are placed at our institution. The continuous invasive blood pressure monitoring is necessary for intraoperative management. Blood pressure changes are sudden and may be drastic. At our institution, patients who have a history of difficulty obtaining peripheral venous access will receive a central venous catheter. Central venous access placement it is at the discretion of the anesthesiology team. Additionally, the interventionalists can place a femoral venous sheath for central venous access, if necessary. However, femoral venous access sheaths are routinely removed before exiting the operating room. Vasopressor agents are connected to the intravenous circuit in preparation for the potential of acute hemodynamic instability. Pulmonary artery catheters are not routinely placed unless a patient-specific concern arises.

PROCEDURE

Before the start of the procedure, multiple safety checks must be completed, including the availability of a dedicated perfusionist with a cardiopulmonary bypass machine as well as a cardiac surgeon on standby. Once all teams are ready, femoral artery and vein access may begin. Local anesthetic is delivered at bilateral groin sites in preparation for venous and arterial sheath insertion. Surgical access might be necessary if percutaneous access is not possible. While accessing the femoral vessels, careful attention to hemodynamics is necessary. Often, patients present with calcified and diseased vessels placing them at high risk for rupture or dissection. If instability occurs upon entry, aggressive volume and pharmacologic resuscitation are necessary until hemorrhage is controlled.[15]

Femoral venous access is obtained for introducing a transvenous right ventricular pacing lead.[31] Next, femoral arteries are accessed. One artery will be the entry site for the delivery system and balloon catheter. A pigtail catheter will be placed in the opposite femoral artery for the aortogram. During either a transapical or direct aortic TAVR with severe femoral disease, the pigtail catheter may be placed in the radial or brachial artery. With endovascular catheters, the patient is at risk for tamponade via chamber perforation. This can be detected by an increasing central venous pressure, if available, decreasing systemic blood pressure, or direct visualization on TEE. If suspected, an immediate pericardiocentesis should be performed to drain the tamponade causing effusion.[32]

If necessary, balloon valvuloplasty can dilate the native aortic valve. This dilation allows for better positioning of the prosthesis especially in patients with critical aortic stenosis, and it improves cardiac output. Fluoroscopy is necessary for exact positioning of the balloon. Before balloon inflation, rapid ventricular pacing at 160 to 200 beat/min is used to prevent balloon migration by ceasing cardiac output. After balloon deflation, rapid pacing is terminated and some patients may require supportive treatment to help recover blood pressure.[33] A bolus dose of phenylephrine will help to restore coronary perfusion. This bolus is critical, and if perfusion pressure unable to be restored with pharmacologic agents such as vasopressin, phenylephrine, or epinephrine, emergent cardiopulmonary bypass must be considered to restore perfusion.

Next, the team will start positioning the prosthesis. The delivery device, which was once much bigger than the current 14-Fr system, is placed in the femoral artery. In a retrograde fashion, it is passed to the ascending aorta and carefully positioned at the native annulus with fluoroscopy and TEE (if available). This aspect of the procedure requires great vigilance because numerous complications may occur at this step, including valve migration into the distal aorta or left ventricle, excessive perivalvular leak, or coronary ostial obstruction.[34] Once the valve is positioned using fluoroscopy, rapid ventricular pacing is again used for deployment. The prosthesis is deployed once cardiac output has ceased. After deployment, pacing is stopped. Patients usually recover without any intervention. During rapid ventricular pacing, the coronary arteries are not well-perfused, causing the heart to weaken because of ischemia. If the patient does not recover adequately, cardiopulmonary bypass must be initiated emergently. Most patients recover with very little intervention. As the stenosis is relieved, the result is a reduction in left ventricular afterload and oxygen consumption, and the left ventricle is able to now deliver a greater cardiac output.

After valve deployment and recovery of hemodynamics, valve function must be assessed. At our institution, an intraoperative transthoracic echocardiography is done to evaluate for any intravalvular or perivalvular regurgitation. Once the images are reviewed and results are deemed satisfactory, angiography of the femoral and iliac arteries are performed to assess any vascular complication, such as dissection or perforation. If the patient's condition remains satisfactory, the delivery system and sheaths are removed. The femoral arteries are either surgically repaired or, if percutaneously accessed, an endovascular device may be used for closure.

If a general anesthetic was used, the patient should be prepped for extubation if bleeding and hemodynamics are stable after deployment and sheath removal. Antiemetics and reversal for muscle relaxants should be administered once patient is considered safe for extubation. Patients should be warmed before extubating. This may be a challenge because the patient's chest and groin are all included in the preparation, leaving no room for a warming blanket.

Sedation allows for continuous neurologic monitoring. After valve deployment, patients should be assessed for possible signs of any neurologic injury such as stroke. However, clinical signs for a stroke will not be evident if the patient is under general anesthesia until after extubation. Immediate diagnostic imaging should be considered if a stroke is suspected.

Another complication seen with postvalve deployment is heart block. Heart block is more common with TAVR than SAVR. Heart block may occur immediately after deployment or days later. Heart block may be immediately treated with temporary pacing, but if persistent, the patient will require a permanent pacemaker.[35]

At our institution, patients may be transferred to the postanesthesia care unit rather than the intensive care unit if stable and extubated.

TAVR is currently more than just an option for those who are deemed too high risk for SAVR. TAVR was recently approved for moderate risk and is currently being evaluated for low-risk patients. TAVR will likely become the standard of care as the number performed every year grows. The procedure will continue to evolve and become even safer than it is now. Recently, there have been case reports of same-day discharge for certain patients who meet specific criteria.

ENDOVASCULAR EDGE-TO-EDGE MITRAL VALVE REPAIR PROCEDURE

In certain patients, mitral regurgitation can be treated in the CCL via a percutaneous approach. In 2013, the FDA approved an alternative to mitral regurgitation repair surgery, endovascular edge to edge mitral valve repair, the MitraClip.[36] Patients who are at increased risk such those with advanced liver disease, previous heart surgery, advanced age, and poor left ventricular function now have a less invasive option.[37]

Additionally, the mitral valve clip procedure has been used to help alleviate systolic anterior leaflet motion in patients with obstructive hypertrophic cardiomyopathy.[38] Although this approach is an alternative option for patients who were denied surgery, some patients may not be a candidate for the mitral clip valve procedure (**Box 1**).

Because the MitraClip procedure requires TEE and careful manipulation of catheters, these patients are placed under general anesthesia and intubated. A complete preoperative evaluation must be done, because these patients are usually too sick or frail for surgical mitral valve intervention. After a careful evaluation, standard ASA monitors along with defibrillating pads are placed on the patient. Before induction of general anesthesia, an invasive continuous arterial blood pressure monitor is recommended. General anesthesia should be induced with careful attention to blood pressure stability, because these patients have marginal left ventricular function. An endotracheal tube is necessary because TEE is essential to the success of the procedure. Additional large peripheral or central intravenous access should be obtained.

The procedure itself involves the interventionalists accessing the femoral vein and directing their catheters to the right atrium. Using TEE as guidance, an intentional puncture through the intraatrial septum allows access to the left atrium. Once in the left atrium, interventionalists, again under TEE and fluoroscopy guidance, pass the clip into the left ventricle through the mitral valve. The clip is then opened and pulled through the mitral valve toward the left atrium attaching to both the anterior and posterior leaflets. Once in a satisfactory position, the clip is closed essentially attaching a portion of the anterior and posterior leaflet together reestablishing leaflet coaptation, comparable with an Alfieri repair or double orifice mitral valve repair.[39]

Endovascular edge-to-edge repair has proven to reduce mitral valve regurgitation with improved functional status, especially in those with severe regurgitation. Because cardiopulmonary bypass is avoided and open heart surgery is not necessary, recovery times are much shorter. However, surgical mitral valve surgery has proven to be more effective in the long term, and remains the standard of care for correcting mitral regurgitation. Patients who are high risk for open heart surgery with symptomatic severe mitral regurgitation now have an option to help correct their valvular dysfunction.[39]

LEFT ATRIAL APPENDAGE CLOSURE DEVICE

Atrial fibrillation is the most common sustained cardiac arrhythmia, affecting more than 6 million people in the United States. Atrial contraction is lost, which leads to

---

Box 1
Contraindications for the *MitraClip* device

Rheumatic mitral valve disease or mitral stenosis
　Mitral valve area <4 cm^2
　Transmitral gradient >5 mm Hg

Femoral venous, inferior vena cava, or intracardiac thrombus

Mitral valve endocarditis

Intolerance to procedural anticoagulation

Intolerance to antiplatelet therapy (necessary after the procedure)

Life expectancy less than 1 year

Data from Abbott. *MitraClip* Clip Delivery System. Available at: http://www.abbottvascular.com/docs/ifu/structural_heart/eIFU_MitraClip.pdf. Accessed July 26 2017.

abnormal flow or stasis. Stagnant blood in the left atrium places the patient at an increased risk for developing a thrombus, which may potentially embolize to the brain resulting in a stroke. For nonvalvular atrial fibrillation, the left atrial appendage is the most common site of thrombus development.[40] Based on the presence or absence of numerous risk factors for stroke, chronic anticoagulation might be necessary to minimize the risk of neurologic injury. Chronic anticoagulation such as warfarin, or newer agents such as direct thrombin or factor Xa inhibitors, are used. However, some patients, although they are at high risk for a stroke, are unable tolerate chronic anticoagulation therapy and require an alternative option.[41]

Mechanically removing or suturing the left atrial appendage is an option usually performed during mitral valve surgery. This very invasive procedure requires placing the patient on cardiopulmonary bypass. Some patients will not be eligible for this option because of the increased risk owing to multiple comorbidities. Additionally, surgical closure of the left atrial appendage may be incomplete, requiring the patient to remain anticoagulated after sternotomy and cardiopulmonary bypass.[42]

A newer technology has emerged as an alternative to anticoagulation for some patients without having to undergo invasive surgery. A percutaneous left atrial occlusion device is now an alternative for patients with nonvalvular atrial fibrillation. The device consists of a Nitinol plug with a fabric component that will occlude the left atrial appendage to prevent a thrombus from forming.[43,44]

Patients should undergo a complete preoperative evaluation. Anticoagulation status should be evaluated with the patient and appropriate laboratory tests such as the International Normalized Ration, prothrombin time, and partial thromboplastin time should be reviewed.

Standard ASA monitors should be applied and a radial arterial catheter for continuous blood pressure monitoring is recommended. As an alternative, a femoral arterial catheter can be placed by the interventionalist. General anesthesia is recommended, because TEE is necessary for positioning the device within the appendage.

Femoral venous access is obtained. The left atrium is accessed by an intraatrial septum puncture guided under fluoroscopy and TEE. Once in the left atrium, measurements are obtained to ensure that the appropriate device is deployed into the left atrial appendage. After deployment, the appendage is assessed again, looking for any residual flow. Once completed, patients are extubated. If the patient is hemodynamically stable, an bed in the intensive care unit is not required at our institution.

CLOSING

Technology is evolving very quickly. More patients have become eligible for procedures to treat cardiac diseases without having to undergo major surgery. Although recent advances in catheter-based therapies afford very sick patients an opportunity at finding relief, these advances will ultimately change our treatment paradigm as the technology evolves and becomes available to everyone. Overall, patients undergoing percutaneous catheter-based therapy will experience faster recovery, shorter durations of hospital stay, and a smaller surgical scar. However, clinicians must remain vigilant; hemodynamic instability can occur at any time. Most patients currently eligible for these procedures often present with multiple comorbidities that deemed them as inoperable surgical candidates. If a complication does arise and more invasive intervention is necessary, the anesthesiologist must be immediately available for resuscitation and aiding in the process of placing the patient on cardiopulmonary bypass, if necessary.

REFERENCES

1. Smith CR, Leon MB, Mack MJ, et al. Transcatheter versus surgical aortic-valve replacement in high-risk patients. N Engl J Med 2011;364(23):2187–98.
2. Leon MB, Smith CR, Mack MJ, et al. Transcatheter or surgical aortic-valve replacement in intermediate-risk patients. N Engl J Med 2016;374(17):1609–20.
3. Leon MB, Smith CR, Mack M, et al. Transcatheter aortic-valve implantation for aortic stenosis in patients who cannot undergo surgery. N Engl J Med 2010; 363(17):1597–607.
4. Nishimura RA, Otto CM, Bonow RO, et al. 2017 AHA/ACC focused update of the 2014 AHA/ACC guideline for the management of patients with valvular heart disease: a report of the American College of Cardiology/American Heart Association Task Force on Clinical Practice Guidelines. J Am Coll Cardiol 2017;135(25): e1159–95.
5. Grover FL, Vemulapalli S, Carroll JD, et al. 2016 annual report of the Society of Thoracic Surgeons/American College of Cardiology transcatheter valve therapy registry. J Am Coll Cardiol 2017;69(10):1215–30.
6. Makkar RR, Fontana GP, Jilaihawi H, et al. Transcatheter aortic-valve replacement for inoperable severe aortic stenosis. N Engl J Med 2012;366(18):1696–704.
7. Adams DH, Popma JJ, Reardon MJ, et al. Transcatheter aortic-valve replacement with a self-expanding prosthesis. N Engl J Med 2014;370(19):1790–8.
8. Reardon MJ, Van Mieghem NM, Popma JJ, et al. Surgical or transcatheter aortic-valve replacement in intermediate-risk patients. N Engl J Med 2017;376(14): 1321–31.
9. Toggweiler S, Gurvitch R, Leipsic J, et al. Percutaneous aortic valve replacement: vascular outcomes with a fully percutaneous procedure. J Am Coll Cardiol 2012; 59(2):113–8.
10. Gotzmann M, Korten M, Bojara W, et al. Long-term outcome of patients with moderate and severe prosthetic aortic valve regurgitation after transcatheter aortic valve implantation. Am J Cardiol 2012;110(10):1500–6.
11. Kodali SK, Williams MR, Smith CR, et al. Two-year outcomes after transcatheter or surgical aortic-valve replacement. N Engl J Med 2012;366(18):1686–95.
12. Tamburino C, Capodanno D, Ramondo A, et al. Incidence and predictors of early and late mortality after transcatheter aortic valve implantation in 663 patients with severe aortic stenosis. Circulation 2011;123(3):299–308.
13. Hahn RT, Pibarot P, Stewart WJ, et al. Comparison of transcatheter and surgical aortic valve replacement in severe aortic stenosis: a longitudinal study of echocardiography parameters in cohort A of the PARTNER trial (placement of aortic transcatheter valves). J Am Coll Cardiol 2013;61(25):2514–21.
14. Pibarot P, Weissman NJ, Stewart WJ, et al. Incidence and sequelae of prosthesis-patient mismatch in transcatheter versus surgical valve replacement in high-risk patients with severe aortic stenosis: a PARTNER trial cohort–a analysis. J Am Coll Cardiol 2014;64(13):1323–34.
15. Van Mieghem NM, Tchetche D, Chieffo A, et al. Incidence, predictors, and implications of access site complications with transfemoral transcatheter aortic valve implantation. Am J Cardiol 2012;110:1361–7.
16. American Society of Anesthesiologists Task Force on Sedation and Analgesia by Non-Anesthesiologists. Practice guidelines for sedation and analgesia by non-anesthesiologists. Anesthesiology 2002;96:1004–17.
17. American Society of Anesthesiologists. Continuum of depth of sedation: definition of general anesthesia and levels of sedation/analgesia.

18. Das S, Ghosh S. Monitored anesthesia care: an overview. J Anesthesiol Clin Pharmacol 2015;31:27–9.
19. Petridis FD, Savini C, Castelli A, et al. Awake transapical aortic valve implantation. Interact Cardiovasc Thorac Surg 2012;14:673–4.
20. Mukherjee C, Walther T, Borger MA, et al. Awake transapical aortic valve implantation using thoracic epidural anesthesia. Ann Thorac Surg 2009;88:992–4.
21. Poltak JM, Cobey FC, Augoustides JG, et al. Paravertebral analgesia in transapical transcatheter aortic valve replacement. Heart Lung Vessel 2015;7:91.
22. Giri J: Moderate vs. General anesthesia for transcatheter aortic valve replacement: an STS/ACC transcatheter valve therapy registry analysis. Society for Cardiovascular Angiography and Interventions Scientific. Sessions, Orlando, FL, May 6, 2016.
23. Bergmann L, Kahlert P, Eggebrecht H, et al. Transfemoral aortic valve implantation under sedation and monitored anaesthetic care—a feasibility study. Anaesthesia 2011;66:977–82.
24. Frohlich GM, Lansky AJ, Webb J, et al. Local versus general anesthesia for transcatheter aortic valve implantation (TAVR)–systematic review and meta-analysis. BMC Med 2014;12:41.
25. Fassa AA, Mazighi M, Himbert D, et al. Successful endovascular stroke rescue with retrieval of an embolized calcium fragment after transcatheter aortic valve replacement. Circ Cardiovasc Interv 2014;7:125–6.
26. Anuwatworn A, Raizada A, Kelly S, et al. Stroke with valve tissue embolization during transcatheter aortic valve replacement treated with endovascular intervention. JACC Cardiovasc Interv 2015;8:1261–3.
27. Reves JG, Glass P, Lubarsky DA, et al. Intravenous anesthetics. Chapter 26. In: Rd Miller, editor. Miller's anesthesia. 7th edition. Philadelphia: Elsevier Churchill Livingstone; 2009. p. 719–68.
28. Bufton KA, Augoustides JG, Cobey FC. Anesthesia for transfemoral aortic valve replacement in North America and Europe. J Cardiothorac Vasc Anesth 2013;27:46–9.
29. Covello RD, Landoni G, Michev I, et al. Percutaneous aortic valve implantation: the anesthesiologist perspective. HSR Proc Intensive Care Cardiovasc Anesth 2009;1:28–38.
30. Christ M, Sharkova Y, Geldner G, et al. Preoperative and perioperative care for patients with suspected or established aortic stenosis facing noncardiac surgery. Chest 2005;128:2944–53.
31. Webb JG, Pasupati S, Achtem L, et al. Rapid pacing to facilitate transcatheter prosthetic heart valve implantation. Catheter Cardiovasc Interv 2006;68:199–204.
32. Kronzon I, Jelnin V, Ruiz C, et al. Optimal imaging for guiding TAVR: transesophageal or transthoracic echocardiography, or just fluoroscopy? JACC Cardiovasc Imaging 2015;8:361–70.
33. Mehta C, Shebani S, Grech V, et al. How to achieve balloon stability in aortic valvuloplasty using rapid ventricular pacing. Images Paediatr Cardiol 2004;6(4):31–7.
34. Billings FT 4th, Kodali SK, Shanewise JS. Transcatheter aortic valve implantation: anesthetic considerations. Anesth Analg 2009;108(5):1453–62.
35. Ghadimi K, Patel PA, Gutsche JT, et al. Perioperative conduction disturbances after transcatheter aortic valve replacement. J Cardiothorac Vasc Anesth 2013;27:1414–20.
36. Whitlow PL, Feldman T, Pedersen WR. Acute and 12-month results with catheter-based mitral valve leaflet repair: the EVEREST II (endovascular valve edge-to-edge repair) high risk study. J Am Coll Cardiol 2012;59:130–9.

37. Mirabel M, Iung B, Baron G, et al. What are the characteristics of patients with severe, symptomatic, mitral regurgitation who are denied surgery? Eur Heart J 2007;28(11):1358–65.
38. Schäfer U, Frerker C, Thielsen T, et al. Targeting systolic anterior motion and left ventricular outflow tract obstruction in hypertrophic obstructed cardiomyopathy with a MitraClip. EuroIntervention 2015;11(8):942–7.
39. Feldman T, Wasserman H, Herrmann H, et al. Percutaneous mitral valve repair using the edge-to-edge technique: six-month results of the EVEREST phase I clinical trial. J Am Coll Cardiol 2005;46(11):2134–40.
40. Fatkin D, Kelly RP, Feneley MP. Relations between left atrial appendage blood flow velocity, spontaneous echocardiographic contrast and thromboembolic risk in vivo. J Am Coll Cardiol 1994;23:961–9.
41. De Backer O, Arnous S, Ihlemann N, et al. Percutaneous left atrial appendage occlusion for stroke prevention in atrial fibrillation: an update. Open Heart 2014;1: e000020.
42. Aryana A, Bhaskar R. Incomplete surgical ligation of the left atrial appendage—time for a new look at an old problem. Ann Transl Med 2017;5(6):141.
43. Al-Saady NM, Obel OA, Camm AJ. Left atrial appendage: structure, function, and role in thromboembolism. Heart 1999;82:547–54.
44. Möbius-Winkler S, Sandri M, Mangner N, et al. The WATCHMAN left atrial appendage closure device for atrial fibrillation. J Vis Exp 2012;(60):e3671.

Anesthesia in the Electrophysiology Laboratory

Jeff E. Mandel, MD, MS[a],*, William G. Stevenson, MD[b],
David S. Frankel, MD[c]

KEYWORDS

- General anesthesia • Conscious sedation • High-frequent jet ventilation
- Catheter ablation • Programmed stimulation

KEY POINTS

- Sedation remains an important modality in the electrophysiology suite and monitoring for respiratory depression is an essential component.
- Scar-related ventricular tachycardia can typically be induced under general anesthesia; however, more aggressive programmed stimulation is often required.
- In contrast, automatic and triggered arrhythmias, as well as reentrant arrhythmias incorporating the atrioventricular node, are more sensitive to catecholamine state.
- General anesthesia and high-frequency jet ventilation decrease patient movement and thoracic excursion, enhancing contact between the ablation catheter and myocardium, resulting in more durable ablation lesions and improved outcomes.
- Use of mechanical hemodynamic support including percutaneous left ventricular assist devices and extracorporeal membrane oxygenation are increasing in ablation of scar-related ventricular tachycardia.

 Video content accompanies this article at http://www.anesthesiology.
theclinics.com.

INTRODUCTION

The electrophysiology (EP) suite is a foreign, and often foreboding location to many anesthesiologists. Like many non–operating room anesthesia areas, the initial experience in

Disclosures: None.
[a] Department of Anesthesiology and Critical Care, Perelman School of Medicine, University of Pennsylvania, 3400 Spruce Street, Philadelphia, PA 19104, USA; [b] Electrophysiology Section, Cardiovascular Division, Brigham and Women's Hospital, 75 Francis Street, Boston, MA 02115, USA; [c] Electrophysiology Section, Cardiovascular Division, Perelman School of Medicine, University of Pennsylvania, 3400 Spruce Street, Philadelphia, PA 19104, USA
* Corresponding author. Hospital of the University of Pennsylvania, 7003 Dulles, 3400 Spruce Street, Philadelphia, PA 19104.
E-mail address: mandelj@uphs.upenn.edu

Anesthesiology Clin 35 (2017) 641–654
http://dx.doi.org/10.1016/j.anclin.2017.07.009   **anesthesiology.theclinics.com**
1932-2275/17/© 2017 Elsevier Inc. All rights reserved.

the EP suite was with shorter procedures performed under conscious sedation (CS), and the value of greater tailoring of the sedation/anesthesia by anesthesiologists was not perceived until practice patterns had already been established. It is not surprising, then, that the reference therapy for studies that assess the impact of anesthetic techniques is most frequently CS. This impact is not always positive; muscle relaxants may preclude identification of the course of the phrenic nerve, rendering it susceptible to ablation injury; anesthetics may suppress arrhythmias, preventing mapping. Anesthesia can also blunt the hemodynamic adaptation to induced arrhythmias, aggravating hypotension and at the same time impeding assessment of cerebral perfusion, factors that are used to guide the duration that an arrhythmia can be allowed to persist to allow mapping and ablation. Thus, it is important when approaching the EP suite to recognize that conventional anesthesia wisdom derived from experience with surgeons may not be optimal for collaborating with electrophysiologists. It is also important to understand that electrophysiologists follow a different path than surgeons during training, and are not inculcated with the culture of the operating room. It is easy for this difference in expectations to lead to arguments that do not serve the interest of the patient. We attempt to address several areas in which an understanding of the requirements of the procedure can enhance care.

PREPROCEDURAL PLANNING

Patients undergoing EP procedures span the gamut of possibilities, from a healthy child to a frail octogenarian. Although anesthesiologists are accustomed to tailoring the anesthetic plan to the level of pain anticipated for the procedure, many EP procedures are minimally invasive, and pain is not the primary reason for involvement of anesthesia providers. It is, therefore, important in planning the anesthetic management to understand the particular arrhythmia.

A commonly performed procedure in EP is placement of an implantable cardiac device (or pacemaker). Many patients can tolerate placement of transvenous devices with minimal sedation, and many centers no longer routinely perform defibrillation threshold testing. When this is needed, a period of sedation or general anesthesia is typically used for cardioversion/defibrillation. More recently, subcutaneous defibrillators have become available, requiring more extensive dissection and tunneling, and general anesthesia is required in most cases. Regional anesthesia may be a useful adjunct during device implantation.

Catheter ablation is the other major category of procedures. Achieving the procedural goal of identifying and ablating the arrhythmia requires consideration of factors that may influence its inducibility and procedural tolerance. Arrhythmias typically originate either from a small focus or larger reentry circuits. Focal arrhythmias are usually due to abnormal automaticity (although small reentry circuits are sometimes encountered) and are more commonly seen in structurally normal hearts. These are referred to as idiopathic; ectopic atrial tachycardia, idiopathic premature ventricular beats, and idiopathic ventricular tachycardia (VT) are common examples. Focal atrial tachycardias may occur after catheter ablation for atrial fibrillation, and focal VTs can arise from diseased Purkinje tissue (fascicular automatic tachycardia). Focal arrhythmias are targeted for ablation by identifying the site of earliest activation during the arrhythmia by moving a catheter across the cardiac chamber of origin during the arrhythmia and plotting the activation time on a 3-dimensional reconstruction of the chamber in an electroanatomic mapping system. Successful ablation of these arrhythmias requires that the arrhythmia be provoked and allowed to persist long enough to be mapped; once mapped, the focus can often be ablated anatomically. Most idiopathic arrhythmias are well-tolerated hemodynamically and rarely require cardioversion. Unfortunately, arrhythmias owing to abnormal automaticity can be exquisitely sensitive to autonomic tone and may be completely suppressed under sedation. In such cases, success depends on the ability of the team to obtain patient cooperation without resorting to excessive use of sedatives and anesthetics, as will be addressed in subsequent sections. Occasionally, idiopathic VT can lead to rates exceeding 250 beats/min, limiting the time that can be spent mapping and potentially requiring administration of vasoconstrictors or urgent cardioversion. The combination of an arrhythmia that is only provokable in the unsedated state and which is also hemodynamically unstable poses a particular challenge.

Reentrant arrhythmias may arise from ventricular or supraventricular locations. Ventricular arrhythmias tend to occur in structurally abnormal hearts, and may be relatively insensitive to autonomic tone. Paroxysmal supraventricular tachycardias, such as atrioventricular (AV) nodal reentry or AV reentry traversing an accessory pathway tend to arise in structurally normal hearts and depend on AV nodal conduction, which is very sensitive to autonomic tone. Conversely, atrial flutter is due to a large reentry circuit, and is typically interrupted by a line of ablation between the inferior vena cava and the tricuspid annulus. Although anesthesia can impair the inducibility of many supraventricular reentrant arrhythmias, this can generally be overcome by administration of beta-agonists, and occasionally atropine. Frequently, ablation targets are identified anatomically for atrial flutter and AV nodal reentry, or during sinus or paced rhythm for an accessory pathway, and extensive mapping during the arrhythmia is usually not required. Supraventricular arrhythmias are usually hemodynamically stable. Thus, fewer constraints are placed on the anesthesia plan.

The ablation approach to atrial fibrillation varies among centers, but is largely anatomically guided, involving electrical isolation of the antral aspect of the pulmonary veins with either radiofrequency ablation or cryoablation. Because extensive ablation is required and control of patient motion can be important, general anesthesia is a common option. If automatic foci are sought as triggers of AF, this is usually done by administering high doses of isoproterenol.

Although ventricular reentrant tachycardias are relatively unaffected by autonomic tone, they are more frequently associated with structurally abnormal hearts, and present significant challenges owing to hemodynamic instability. Although the arrhythmia is usually inducible under anesthesia, baroreflex responses to hypotension during induced tachycardia may be impaired. An induced VT at 150 beats/min that is hemodynamically tolerated when the patient is conscious may produce persistent hypotension during anesthesia, requiring prompt termination and limiting the time that can be spent in VT for mapping. The concern is often magnified by depressed ventricular function, which is usually present in patients with scar-related VT. This population is also often at risk for myocardial ischemia from coronary artery disease and other comorbidities are often present. However, many of these arrhythmias can now be targeted for ablation by identifying the regions of scar and potential reentry circuits during stable sinus or paced rhythm, and targeting these regions for ablation. This approach, referred to as substrate mapping, markedly reduces the need to induce VT, which may be done only at the beginning and end of the procedure. As discussed elsewhere in this article, scar-related VT increasingly is being managed with circulatory support.

ANTICIPATED CHALLENGES

The EP laboratory is remarkable for its diversity of patients and procedures, as well as challenges that vary with the patient. Some arrhythmias require ablation adjacent to a phrenic nerve. The right phrenic nerve can be at risk for damage during ablation near the right pulmonary veins, superior vena cava, and lateral right atrium. The left phrenic nerve can be injured from ablation in or near the left atrial appendage, or over the epicardium of the left ventricle. The courses of the phrenic nerves are variable, and identified by pacing from the ablation catheter and observing for diaphragmatic stimulation. It is, therefore, important that paralytics are not used in these patients.

Some arrhythmia targets require an approach from the epicardium. This is usually achieved by subxiphoid pericardial puncture, using the Sosa technique.[1] Because the pericardium may have minimal fluid, this can be a challenging procedure with a risk of puncture or laceration of the right ventricle and cardiac tamponade. Brief periods of apnea can potentially facilitate access. Apnea can also be useful to facilitate catheter stability during ablation at sites near a critical structure, such as the AV node. The important role of high-frequency jet ventilation (HFJV) in providing extended periods free from respiratory motion is discussed elsewhere in this article.

The anesthesiologist may be the first provider to encounter signs of a developing problem, with increasing vasopressor requirements or a change in ventilatory parameters. Cardiac perforation and tamponade occurs in 0.5% to 1% of procedures. Significant bleeding into the retroperitoneum or thigh from femoral access sites can occur with little superficially visible evidence, particularly in obese patients. Many ablation procedures, particularly those done for AF, are done with the patient on systemic anticoagulation with warfarin or a direct acting anticoagulant, to which intravenous heparin is added. Prompt recognition of these issues is crucial. Maintaining rapport with the EP team throughout the procedure and discussing physiologic changes is important for early recognition of problems and is facilitated by a discussion of potential challenges before the procedure.

Intracardiac ultrasound imaging is used in many laboratories to aid in the creation of anatomic shells for mapping, guide transseptal puncture, and monitor ventricular function and potential complications, including cardiac tamponade. When concern arises, taking a moment in the midst of the procedure to position the ultrasound probe to assess, and hopefully exclude, an emerging problem such as cardiac tamponade, can be helpful.

SEDATION

Much of the initial experience in EP was obtained with proceduralist-directed sedation, and many electrophysiologists feel strongly that this is sufficient for most procedures.[2] Increasingly, however, anesthesia providers are constant fixtures in the EP laboratory, and sedation practices are changing.

The 3 mechanisms of tachyarrhythmia include reentry, automaticity, and triggered activity. Typically, automatic and triggered arrhythmias are catecholamine sensitive, and are more difficult to initiate under general anesthesia in comparison to sedation. Although the administration of agents such as isoproterenol will typically prevail, prolonged administration of isoproterenol to sedated patients may be unpleasant. Reentrant arrhythmias may also be suppressed by sedatives and anesthetic agents. It is important to discuss the plan for sedation with the electrophysiologist. It is not unusual in our institutions to obtain bladder and vascular access under deep sedation, mapping under minimal sedation, and then induce general anesthesia once an ablation target has been identified.

During long procedures, sedation may lead to respiratory depression and obstruction. Obstruction during EP procedures may be problematic, because the anesthesia provider's hands are exposed to fluoroscopy when performing jaw thrust. The Jaw Elevation Device (Hypnoz Therapeutic Devices, Cardiff-by-the-Sea, CA) can be useful in this setting. Narron and colleagues[3] audited quality improvement data for sedation cases using the device and found that in 9 of 10 cases, desaturation could be avoided. Davila-Moriel and colleauges[4] found that 20 of 28 patients experiencing airway obstruction could be managed solely with the device. In our experience, the device can be useful in avoiding transitioning to laryngeal mask airway (LMA) or intubation, and reduces exposure of anesthesia personnel to fluoroscopy, an underappreciated problem.[5]

Appropriate monitoring of patients undergoing prolonged sedation is an important consideration. The pulse oximeter is an unreliable measure of respiratory depression, particularly when supplemental oxygen is administered, because it will mask decreases in minute ventilation until the patient "falls off the cliff."[6] Although capnography has been advocated as a means of detecting the onset of apnea before desaturation, a prospective study of procedural sedation using propofol and ketamine in 63 patients breathing room air found only a weak correlation between abnormal capnography and desaturation.[7] Indeed, none of the patients who met the criteria for both abnormal capnometry and desaturation experienced abnormal capnometry before the onset of desaturation; the only finding that preceded desaturation was a decrease in end tidal CO_2 (presumably attributable to shallow breathing). In a prospective study of 427 patients undergoing procedural sedation with propofol, adding capnography to standard monitoring did not significantly reduce the incidence of desaturation. Although a metaanalysis of outcomes with capnography found that it was associated with a decrease in the frequency of desaturation, there was no association between capnography and any other endpoint, such as assisted ventilation or jaw thrust.[8] Although capnography may be a useful adjunct in some settings, it can be associated with a high rate of false alarms and is expensive to acquire and maintain. The cost–benefit ratio of capnography may soon be exceeded by newer technologies that are being incorporated into standard monitors. One such example is the Masimo Respiratory Acoustic Monitor (Masimo, Irvine CA), which has been shown to accurately track changes in respiratory rate in operating room conditions.[9] Masimo has also developed the Oxygen Reserve Index, a measurement that can assess the decrease in P_{AO_2} between 200 and 100 mm Hg (when oxygen saturation is >98%).[10] Medtronic (North Haven, CT) has demonstrated the ability to accurately recover respiratory rates from amplitude modulation of the pulse oximeter waveform,[11] and presented data indicating that respiratory modulation of the plethysmograph can assess increases in respiratory effort.[12]

New monitors may provide the clinician more useful information. Transcutaneous monitoring of CO_2 has become increasingly practical owing to the introduction of digital monitors (SenTec, Therwil, Arlasheim, BL, Switzerland). Transcutaneous measurements were found to correlate consistently with arterial samples in respiratory failure patients undergoing noninvasive ventilation.[13] The ExSpiron respiratory volume monitor (Respiratory Motion, Waltham, MA) has been demonstrated to reliably estimate minute ventilation during procedural sedation[14] and to provide information on changes in respiratory status more quickly than capnography in spontaneously breathing subjects.[15] All of these measures are significant improvements over simply waiting for the pulse oximeter to declare a crisis; by the time a crisis occurs, heroic measures may be required. The newer monitors offer more than simply informing us when we have given too much sedation and need to rescue; transcutaneous CO_2 has been incorporated into a model of respiratory response to propofol-remifentanil sedation.[16] It is quite easy to use the SenTec monitor to titrate remifentanil to a desired increase in transcutaneous CO_2 in advance of a planned noxious stimulus; in the future, it is quite possible that we will have physiologic closed loop control systems that maintain sedation at a specified level of respiratory depression in the face of changing levels of procedural stimulation.

Infusions of propofol may be used for prolonged deep sedation, but afford limited advantages for arrhythmia inducibility in comparison with general anesthesia, and carry significant risk of respiratory depression and hypotension.[17] The effects of propofol on cardiac EP are myriad,[18] and it is difficult to predict whether it will be advantageous or deleterious in any given situation. Propofol has been associated with termination of supraventricular tachycardia[19] and VT storm.[20]

Etomidate has been advocated for brief sedation for cardioversion[21] and defibrillator threshold testing,[22] but the incidence of myoclonus with etomidate may interfere with immediate interpretation of the electrocardiograph. In a Cochrane review of anesthetic techniques for cardioversion,[23] it was noted that the quality of evidence supporting any technique was low, and that any of the agents used in comparisons would be adequate. Ultimately, the choice of dose and rate of administration may have more bearing on outcome that the actual drug chosen.

The selective α_2 agonist dexmedetomidine has the advantage of less respiratory depression in comparison with propofol.[24] Dexmedetomidine has considerable potential to suppress reentrant supraventricular tachycardias,[25,26] although these effects may be countered by coadministration of ketamine.[27] Ketamine was shown to increase atrial conduction, heart rate, and blood pressure in comparison with propofol,[28] although this did not alter inducibility of supraventricular tachycardia. The combination of dexmedetomidine and ketamine has been demonstrated to reduce the frequency of transient obstruction during therapeutic bronchoscopy in comparison to fentanyl/midazolam sedation. The combination of dexmedetomidine and remifentanil was also demonstrated to provide deeper sedation, less respiratory depression, better analgesia, and greater electrophysiologist satisfaction ratings compared with the combination of midazolam and remifentanil.[29] An advantage of dexmedetomidine is that it is very difficult to create unintended general anesthesia with the drug; patients remain arousable and cooperative.

Another option is remifentanil analgosedation, which offers the advantages of preserved arrhythmia inducibility and hemodynamic stability, while maintaining the ability to assess neurologic examination during VT.[30] The ability to use remifentanil during groin access and discontinue it with near complete clearance in less than 30 minutes makes this agent attractive for arrhythmias that are easily suppressed by other agents.

GENERAL ANESTHESIA

General anesthesia offers advantages for the patient and anesthesia provider, but may inhibit induction of some arrhythmias and removes the ability to monitor neurologic status during sustained VT. Although it is tempting to believe that because halothane increased ventricular ectopy in the presence of epinephrine in normal hearts, that it would be useful for induction of reentrant tachycardias, in a postinfarction model of reentrant VT, halothane, enflurane, and isoflurane[31] have actually been demonstrated to inhibit arrhythmia induction. Desflurane and sevoflurane[32] reduced the rate of spontaneous ventricular ectopy in this model, although to a lesser extent than halothane. Sevoflurane has been shown to prolong accessory pathway effective refractory period in comparison with propofol.[33] The prolongation of QTc interval induced by sevoflurane has been shown to resolve by switching to propofol infusion in as little as 15 minutes.[34] Nof and colleagues[35] demonstrated that most VTs induced before induction of general anesthesia could still be induced under general anesthesia, although often more aggressive programmed stimulation was required. Although general anesthesia has been advocated as safer for management of complex abla-tions, a review of epicardial VT ablation cases found no difference in complications or procedural success, in comparison with sedation.[36] Thus, the choice of general anesthesia or sedation should be tailored to the arrhythmia being treated and under-lying patient substrate.

BETA-ADRENERGIC STIMULATION FOR ARRHYTHMIA INDUCTION AND TESTING

Initiation of catecholamine-sensitive arrhythmias can be facilitated by infusion of isoproterenol. Isoproterenol is commonly used during atrial fibrillation ablation to identify arrhythmia triggers and induce pulmonary vein reconnections. Although gen-eral anesthesia may suppress sympathetically mediated arrhythmias, isoproterenol has been shown to usually prevail, although much higher doses of phenylephrine are often required to support blood pressure.[37] Isoproterenol affects more than the heart; O'Neil and colleagues[38] studied 20 patients undergoing isoproterenol stimula-tion tests and found significant increases in BIS (mean, 24.6) accompanied with spontaneous movement in 60% and response to command in 50% of patients. Although no patients experienced recall, the study was not powered to detect this endpoint. The ability of beta-adrenergic agonists to cause arousal during anesthesia is well-known, although the mechanisms are not completely understood. Isoproter-enol typically produces hypotension, and it might seem counterintuitive to increase the depth of anesthesia concomitantly with its administration. The use of processed electroencephalography may be useful in titrating the depth of anesthesia in this setting.

When performing isoproterenol stimulation tests, a balance must be struck between the effects of isoproterenol and phenylephrine. The interquartile range of isoproterenol doses required to induce AF triggers was reported to be 20 to 111 μg by Mountanto-nakis and colleagues[37]; phenylephrine doses ranged from 52 to 600 μg. Isoproterenol has marked interindividual variability in both pharmacokinetics and pharmacody-namics,[39] so there is no fixed ratio of isoproterenol and phenylephrine that will work in all patients. A useful strategy is usually to change phenylephrine administration 10 to 20 seconds before changing isoproterenol and adjust the ratio based on blood pressure response. When doing this, it is essential to minimize propagation delays in the infusion system by infusing as close to the patient as possible. If ganged stop-cocks are used, place the phenylephrine closer to the patient to reduce the potential for carrying a bolus of isoproterenol along with a bolus of phenylephrine.[40]

EFFECTS OF RESPIRATORY MOTION ON CATHETER STABILITY

During ablation procedures, stable contact between the ablation catheter and tar-geted tissue is essential as radiofrequency energy is applied. Poor tissue contact can result in edema and transient cellular injury without permanent destruction of the arrhythmogenic substrate, resulting in long-term arrhythmia recurrence. Excessive force increases the risk of perforation. Although any form of motion can be disruptive, respiratory motion is particularly problematic, especially during pulmonary vein isola-tion (PVI), because this not only moves the heart within the chest, it also changes the diameter of the pulmonary vein ostia.[41] When performing PVI under CS, this motion is difficult to predict, because breathing becomes increasingly chaotic under sedation. Even more problematic is airway obstruction; the Mueller maneuver dramatically en-larges the atria. Although suppression of patient motion is a useful feature of general anesthesia, control of breathing is the major advantage of the technique. This advan-tage was demonstrated in a randomized trial comparing 257 patients with paroxysmal atrial fibrillation assigned to ablation under inhalational anesthesia with positive pressure ventilation (general anesthesia) or CS with fentanyl and midazolam.[42] General anesthesia was associated with shorter procedure times, lower fluoroscopy exposure, and greater freedom from AF after 1.5 years. Additionally, in those patients who experienced a recurrence of AF, patients whose initial PVI was performed under GA had fewer reconnected pulmonary veins than those whose initial PVI was performed under CS. A further reduction in pulmonary motion can be obtained with HFJV. This was demonstrated retrospectively to improve ablation outcomes in 1332 primary AF ablations.[43] Despite baseline characteristics associated with poorer outcomes (greater body mass index, larger left atrial dimension, and more persistent AF), patients managed with HFJV had lower fluoroscopy exposure, fewer acute and chronic pulmonary vein reconnections, and greater freedom from AF at 1 year. Improved catheter stability with HFJV can be appreciated in the supplemental videos. Video 1 shows displacement of the ablation catheter inferiorly during an inspiration under standard GA. In contrast, Video 2 demonstrates stable catheter position throughout under HFJV.

Despite considerable experience with HFJV in recent years, there has not yet been a randomized comparison of HFJV and conventional mechanical ventilation. For most electrophysiologists, the lack of trial data is unimportant; the difference in catheter stability is immediately obvious. From a logistical standpoint, procedures are either performed under CS without an anesthesia provider, or under GA with an anesthesia provider. Thus, the question frequently posed by anesthesiologists unfamiliar with HFJV is, "Why not just turn up the rate on the conventional ventilator?" To understand the reason, a brief discussion of the physics of ventilation is required.

During conventional ventilation, flow in the trachea is principally plug flow. Although laminar flow occurs at the mucosal surface, the advancing waveform is largely flat, and there is limited mixing between the incoming fresh gas and the alveolar gas. To remove CO_2, the tidal volume must exceed the volume of the trachea, referred to as dead space. As tidal volume decreases, the fraction of ventilation that does not result in CO_2 elimination increases. During HFJV, a narrow stream of gas is emitted from the jet nozzle. This high-velocity jet moves down the core of the airway and undergoes limited mixing with the surrounding gas; during exhalation the same plug flow is seen. This results in a tube within a tube (**Fig. 1**), with relatively low dead space, and is termed *axial dispersion*. This is distinct from *Taylor dispersion*, which is mixing of gas at the leading edge of plug flow. An additional problem with increasing the rate of the conventional ventilator is that the anesthesia circuit is compressible and, as the frequency increases, an increasing fraction of the energy delivered by the ventilator is consumed by the expansion and contraction of the circuit. This results in an overestimation of airway pressure and an underestimation of minute ventilation. At high rates, the end-tidal gas is not truly an alveolar sample, and the gradient between the end-tidal and arterial CO_2 becomes large and variable. Although the sight of familiar phasic waveforms may be comforting, the information contained within becomes unreliable.

Another concern expressed by those unfamiliar with HFJV is the danger of breath stacking—that is, the initiation of a new breath before the lung has completely emptied. These effects are difficult to measure under normal clinical conditions, but lung volume can be estimated using respiratory inductance plethysmography with proper calibration. Passive exhalation is driven by alveolar compliance, and follows the same time course in conventional mechanical ventilation and HFJV (**Fig. 2**). A safety feature of the Monsoon Jet Ventilator (Acutronic Medical Systems, Fabrik im Schifli, Herzel, Switzerland) is pause pressure monitoring. After each breath, the

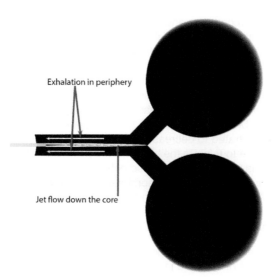

Fig. 1. Axial dispersion during jet ventilation. The inspiratory flow from the jet is restricted to the core of the trachea, while the expiratory flow traverses the periphery.

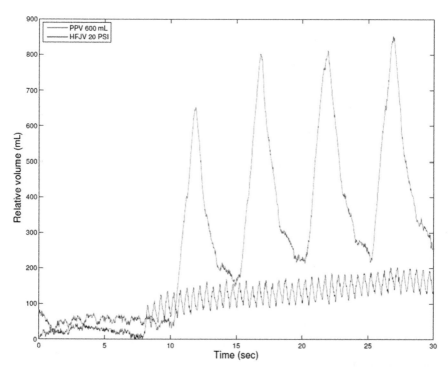

Fig. 2. Thoracic volume measured by respiratory inductance plethysmography under high-frequency jet ventilation at 20 pounds per square inch (*blue*) and positive pressure ventilation at 600 mL tidal volume, each producing similar CO_2 elimination.

pressure in the hose is monitored, and if it does not fall below a specified pressure (eg, 20 cm H_2O) the ventilator alarms and shuts off.

In most patients, HFJV is successful in efficiently removing CO_2 at normal driving pressures, typically 20 to 22 pounds per square inch. In a small subset of patients, CO_2 may be observed to increase. The typical response to this is to increase the driving pressure. Although this will increase the elimination of CO_2, it will also increase intrathoracic pressure, which will decrease venous return, leading to hypotension. Although this may be blamed on the vasoconstrictive effects of hypercarbia, remifentanil has been demonstrated to decrease pulmonary vascular tone.[44] Thus, the more prudent course may be to tolerate the hypercarbia, particularly if no evidence of right ventricular overload is noted on intracardiac echo.

The use of HFJV is increasing in EP laboratories; approximately 50% of sales of the Monsoon Jet Ventilator are now for use in EP suites.

MONITORING BRAIN PERFUSION DURING VENTRICULAR TACHYCARDIA

During ablation of hemodynamically unstable arrhythmias, general anesthesia precludes the assessment of changes in neurologic status. Near-infrared spectroscopy has been advocated as a means for assessing cerebral oxygenation,[45] although the evidence supporting this technique is not strong. Although there is evidence that processed electroencephalography is sensitive to cerebral hypoperfusion states,[46] there are no reports of use of this modality in EP. Given the relatively low volume of cases in which cerebral hypoperfusion is a feature, progress in this area will be slow.

HEMODYNAMIC SUPPORT

When ablating scar-related VT, there is significant risk of acute hemodynamic compromise,[47] which has increased interest in percutaneous mechanical circulatory support.[48] In a prospective crossover study of 20 patients, use of the Impella percutaneous left ventricular assist device (Abiomed, Danvers, MA) was shown to decrease the incidence of cerebral desaturation from 53% to 5%. Use of the Impella

Table 1
Considerations for anesthetic management

Arrhythmia	Need for Inducible Arrhythmia			Potential for Hemodynamic Instability	Sedation May Suppress Arrhythmia	Phrenic Nerve Identification Needed
	Brief	Sustained	None			
Typical atrial flutter	–	–	+	–	–	–
Atypical atrial flutter	+	+	±	–	–	–
Atrial fibrillation	–	–	+	–	+	+
Paroxysmal SVT	+	–	+	–	++	–
Ectopic atrial tachycardia	+	+	–	–	+++	Rarely
Idiopathic focal VT/ PVCs	±	+	±	–	+++	Rarely
Sustained monomorphic VT	±	±	±	+	+	If epicardial

Abbreviations: PVC, premature ventricular contractions; SVT, supraventricular tachycardia; VT, ventricular tachycardia.

percutaneous left ventricular assist device allowed longer mapping times during VT, which allows better identification of ablation targets.[49] Recently, extracorporeal membrane oxygenation has been studied as a primary support technique in patients not otherwise requiring mechanical circulatory support.[50] The use of such measures is in rapid evolution, and although the majority of VT ablation can be managed with vasopressor infusions, the use of mechanical support may become more common, although hemodynamic support has not yet been demonstrated to improve long-term VT-free survival after ablation.

SUMMARY

Several important considerations must be balanced when selecting an anesthetic approach, including patient comfort, arrhythmia inducibility, hemodynamic tolerance, and catheter stability **(Table 1)**. Close communication between the anesthesiologist and electrophysiologist is needed to optimize outcomes.

SUPPLEMENTARY DATA

Supplementary data related to this article can be found online at http://dx.doi.org/10.1016/j.anclin.2017.07.009.

REFERENCES

1. Sosa E, Scanavacca M, d'Avila A, et al. A new technique to perform epicardial mapping in the electrophysiology laboratory. J Cardiovasc Electrophysiol 1996; 7(6):531–6.
2. Gerstein NS, Young A, Schulman PM, et al. Sedation in the electrophysiology laboratory: a multidisciplinary review. J Am Heart Assoc 2016;5(6):e003629.
3. Narron J, Dalal P, Dhar P, et al. Effectiveness of the jaw elevation device in prevention of desaturation during sedation and monitored anesthesia care: a prospective QA audit. In ASA Scientific Sessions. Washington, DC, 2012.
4. Davila-Moriel E, Judd Whiting MD, Tostenrud R. Use of the jaw elevation device in deep sedation. In ASA Scientific Sessions. San Diego, CA, 2015.
5. Andreoli S, Moretti R, Lorini FL, et al. Radiation exposure of an anaesthesiologist in catheterisation and electrophysiological cardiac procedures. Radiat Prot Dosimetry 2016;168(1):76–82.
6. Fu ES, Downs JB, Schweiger JW, et al. Supplemental oxygen impairs detection of hypoventilation by pulse oximetry. Chest 2004;126(5):1552–8.
7. Sivilotti ML, Messenger DW, van Vlymen J, et al. A comparative evaluation of capnometry versus pulse oximetry during procedural sedation and analgesia on room air. CJEM 2010;12(05):397–404.
8. Conway A, Douglas C, Sutherland JR. A systematic review of capnography for sedation. Anaesthesia 2016;71(4):450–4.
9. Atkins JH, Mandel JE. Performance of Masimo rainbow acoustic monitoring for tracking changing respiratory rates under laryngeal mask airway general anesthesia for surgical procedures in the operating room: a prospective observational study. Anesth Analg 2014;119(6):1307–14.
10. Applegate RL, Dorotta IL, Wells B, et al. The relationship between oxygen reserve index and arterial partial pressure of oxygen during surgery. Anesth Analg 2016; 123(3):626–33.

11. Bergese SD, Mestek ML, Kelley SD, et al. Multicenter study validating accuracy of a continuous respiratory rate measurement derived from pulse oximetry: a comparison with capnography. Anesth Analg 2017;124(4):1153–9.

12. Addison PS. Respiratory effort from the photoplethysmogram. Med Eng Phys 2017;41:9–18.

13. Lermuzeaux M, Meric H, Sauneuf B, et al. Superiority of transcutaneous CO_2 over end-tidal CO_2 measurement for monitoring respiratory failure in nonintubated patients: a pilot study. J Crit Care 2016;31(1):150–6.

14. Holley K, MacNabb CM, Georgiadis P, et al. Monitoring minute ventilation versus respiratory rate to measure the adequacy of ventilation in patients undergoing upper endoscopic procedures. J Clin Monit Comput 2016;30(1):33–9.

15. Williams GW, George CA, Harvey BC, et al. A comparison of measurements of change in respiratory status in spontaneously breathing volunteers by the exspiron noninvasive respiratory volume monitor versus the capnostream capnometer. Anesth Analg 2017;124(1):120–6.

16. Hannam JA, Borrat X, Trocóniz IF, et al. Modeling respiratory depression induced by remifentanil and propofol during sedation and analgesia using a continuous noninvasive measurement of pCO_2. J Pharmacol Exp Ther 2016;356(3):563–73.

17. Trentman TL, Fassett SL, Mueller JT, et al. Airway interventions in the cardiac electrophysiology laboratory: a retrospective review. J Cardiothorac Vasc Anesth 2009;23(6):841–5.

18. Liu Q, Kong A-L, Chen R, et al. Propofol and arrhythmias: two sides of the coin. Acta Pharmacol Sin 2011;32(6):817–23.

19. Kannan S, Sherwood N. Termination of supraventricular tachycardia by propofol. Br J Anaesth 2002;88(6):874–5.

20. Burjorjee JE, Milne B. Propofol for electrical storm; a case report of cardioversion and suppression of ventricular tachycardia by propofol. Can J Anaesth 2002; 49(9):973–7.

21. Desai PM, Kane D, Sarkar MS. Cardioversion: what to choose? Etomidate or propofol. Ann Card Anaesth 2015;18(3):306–11.

22. Zgoła K, Kułakowski P, Czepiel A, et al. Haemodynamic effects of etomidate, propofol and electrical shock in patients undergoing implantable cardioverter-defibrillator testing. Kardiol Pol 2014;72(8):707–15.

23. Lewis SR, Nicholson A, Reed SS, et al. Anaesthetic and sedative agents used for electrical cardioversion. Cochrane Database Syst Rev 2015;(3):CD010824.

24. Prachanpanich N, Apinyachon W, Ittichaikulthol W, et al. A comparison of dexmedetomidine and propofol in patients undergoing electrophysiology study. J Med Assoc Thai 2013;96(3):307–11.

25. Chrysostomou C, Morell VO, Wearden P, et al. Dexmedetomidine: therapeutic use for the termination of reentrant supraventricular tachycardia. Congenit Heart Dis 2013;8(1):48–56.

26. Tirotta CF, Nguyen T, Fishberger S, et al. Dexmedetomidine use in patients undergoing electrophysiological study for supraventricular tachyarrhythmias. Paediatr Anaesth 2017;27(1):45–51.

27. Char D, Drover DR, Motonaga KS, et al. The effects of ketamine on dexmedetomidine-induced electrophysiologic changes in children. Paediatr Anaesth 2013;23(10):898–905.

28. Wutzler A, Huemer M, Boldt L-H, et al. Effects of deep sedation on cardiac electrophysiology in patients undergoing radiofrequency ablation of supraventricular tachycardia: impact of propofol and ketamine. Europace 2013;15(7):1019–24.

29. Cho JS, Shim J-K, Na S, et al. Improved sedation with dexmedetomidine-remifentanil compared with midazolam-remifentanil during catheter ablation of atrial fibrillation: a randomized, controlled trial. Europace 2014;16(7):1000–6.

30. Mandel JE, Hutchinson MD, Marchlinski FE. Remifentanil-midazolam sedation provides hemodynamic stability and comfort during epicardial ablation of ventricular tachycardia. J Cardiovasc Electrophysiol 2011;22(4):464–6.

31. Deutsch N, Hantler CB, Tait AR, et al. Suppression of ventricular arrhythmias by volatile anesthetics in a canine model of chronic myocardial infarction. Anesthesiology 1990;72(6):1012–21.

32. Novalija E, Hogan QH, Kulier AH, et al. Effects of desflurane, sevoflurane and halothane on postinfarction spontaneous dysrhythmias in dogs. Acta Anaesthesiol Scand 1998;42(3):353–7.

33. Caldwell JC, Fong C, Muhyaldeen SA. Should sevoflurane be used in the electrophysiology assessment of accessory pathways? Europace 2010;12(9):1332–5.

34. Kleinsasser A, Loeckinger A, Lindner KH, et al. Reversing sevoflurane-associated Q-Tc prolongation by changing to propofol. Anaesthesia 2001;56(3):248–50.

35. Nof E, Reichlin T, Enriquez AD, et al. Impact of general anesthesia on initiation and stability of VT during catheter ablation. Heart Rhythm 2015;12(11):2213–20.

36. Killu AM, Sugrue A, Munger TM, et al. Impact of sedation vs. general anaesthesia on percutaneous epicardial access safety and procedural outcomes. Europace 2016. [Epub ahead of print].

37. Mountantonakis SE, Elkassabany N, Kondapalli L, et al. Provocation of atrial fibrillation triggers during ablation: does the use of general anesthesia affect inducibility? J Cardiovasc Electrophysiol 2015;26(1):16–20.

38. O'Neill DK, Aizer A, Bloom MJ, et al. Isoproterenol increases BIS and arousal during catheter ablation for atrial fibrillation. J Anesth Patient Care 2017;1(2):1–8.

39. Hjemdahl P, Martinsson A, Larsson K. Improvement of the isoprenaline infusion test by plasma concentration measurements. Life Sci 1986;39(7):629–35.

40. Lovich MA, Wakim MG, Wei A, et al. Drug infusion system manifold dead-volume impacts the delivery response time to changes in infused medication doses in vitro and also in vivo in anesthetized swine. Anesth Analg 2013;117(6):1313–8.

41. Ector J, De Buck S, Loeckx D, et al. Changes in left atrial anatomy due to respiration: impact on three-dimensional image integration during atrial fibrillation ablation. J Cardiovasc Electrophysiol 2008;19(8):828–34.

42. Di Biase L, Conti S, Mohanty P, et al. General anesthesia reduces the prevalence of pulmonary vein reconnection during repeat ablation when compared with conscious sedation: results from a randomized study. Heart Rhythm 2011;8(3):368–72.

43. Hutchinson MD, Garcia FC, Mandel JE, et al. Efforts to enhance catheter stability improve atrial fibrillation ablation outcome. Heart Rhythm 2012;10(3):347–53.

44. Kaye AD, Baluch A, Phelps J, et al. An analysis of remifentanil in the pulmonary vascular bed of the cat. Anesth Analg 2006;102(1):118–23.

45. Moerman A, Meert F, De Hert S. Cerebral near-infrared spectroscopy in the care of patients during cardiological procedures: a summary of the clinical evidence. J Clin Monit Comput 2016;30(6):901–9.

46. Cavus E, Meybohm P, Doerges V, et al. Effects of cerebral hypoperfusion on bispectral index: a randomised, controlled animal experiment during haemorrhagic shock. Resuscitation 2010;81(9):1183–9.

47. Santangeli P, Muser D, Zado ES, et al. Acute hemodynamic decompensation during catheter ablation of scar-related ventricular tachycardia: incidence, predictors, and impact on mortality. Circ Arrhythm Electrophysiol 2015;8(1):68–75.

48. Bunch TJ, Mahapatra S, Madhu Reddy Y, et al. The role of percutaneous left ventricular assist devices during ventricular tachycardia ablation. Europace 2012; 14(Suppl 2):ii26–32.
49. Aryana A, Gearoid O'Neill P, Gregory D, et al. Procedural and clinical outcomes after catheter ablation of unstable ventricular tachycardia supported by a percutaneous left ventricular assist device. Heart Rhythm 2014;11(7):1122–30.
50. Sabbag A, Beinart R, Eldar M, et al. Ventricular tachycardia radiofrequency ablation with extracorporeal membrane oxygenation. Interv Cardiol J 2016.

Cardioversions and Transthoracic Echocardiography

Ronak Shah, MD*, Elizabeth Zhou, MD

KEYWORDS

- Atrial fibrillation • Cardioversion • Anesthesia • Sedation
- Transthoracic echocardiography

KEY POINTS

- Anesthesia for transthoracic echocardiography and cardioversions are routinely done outside of the operating room.
- Patients require similar preoperative evaluation as they would for before a surgical procedure.
- A complete check of all necessary supplies and rescue items must be completed before cardioversion or transthoracic echocardiography to ensure patient safety, as most patients will not have a secured airway.
- Appropriate medications for anesthesia should be selected based on patients' comorbidities, and hemodynamic supportive medications, such as phenylephrine, epinephrine, and atropine, should be readily available.

Cardioversion is typically used for conversion of atrial fibrillation and flutter back to normal sinus rhythm. Cardioversion is routinely performed as a non–operating room procedure for which anesthesiologists are requested to provide analgesia and sedation. The anesthetic goals are to provide amnesia of the shock and prevent residual pain. Although these patients often present with other cardiopulmonary comorbidities that will add to the complexity of providing a short effective anesthetic, these patients typically are discharged home after the procedure.

Atrial Flutter

Atrial flutter is a re-entrant circuit in the right atrium. Boundaries for this re-entrant circuit include the tricuspid valve ring and an area of block, which is in the region

Disclosure Statement: The authors have nothing to disclose.
Department of Anesthesiology and Critical Care, Hospital of the University of Pennsylvania, 3400 Spruce Street, Philadelphia, PA 19104, USA
* Corresponding author.
E-mail address: Ronak.Shah@uphs.upenn.edu

Anesthesiology Clin 35 (2017) 655–667
http://dx.doi.org/10.1016/j.anclin.2017.08.002
1932-2275/17/© 2017 Elsevier Inc. All rights reserved.

anesthesiology.theclinics.com

between the venae cavae. A myocardial isthmus of conduction is also present, which is bound by the tricuspid ring and the inferior vena cava, the Eustachian ridge, and the coronary sinus.[1] Atypical atrial scar tissue from a prior atrial incision or around the pulmonary veins can result in atrial flutter.[2] Transthoracic echocardiography (TEE) is the preferred method of evaluation, as it can assess biventricular function and atria size.

Treatment

Treatment goals are centered around ventricular rate control, restoration of sinus rhythm, prevention of recurrent episodes of arrhythmia, and minimizing risk of thromboembolism. Overall, compared with atrial fibrillation, catheter-based ablation is superior to pharmacologic interventions. Cardiologists may consider cardioversion for flutter less than 48 hours in duration or if the patient is hemodynamically unstable.[3]

Atrial Fibrillation

Atrial fibrillation is characterized as a supraventricular tachyarrhythmia with uncoordinated atrial activation and, consequently, ineffective atrial contraction. Atrial fibrillation is the most common sustained cardiac arrhythmia and is associated with a 6-fold increase risk in stroke and 2-fold increase in mortality.[4] Complications associated with atrial fibrillation are related to both loss of atrial contraction and the irregular and rapid ventricular rate. Treatment plans are centered around minimizing risk of embolic events, rate control, and attempting to restore sinus rhythm.

Classification

The 2014 American Heart Association guidelines classify atrial fibrillation from the first detected episode usually presenting for medical attention (**Table 1**). Guidelines describe the persistence of each episode. If the arrhythmia terminates in less than 7 days, it is classified as paroxysmal. If arrhythmia lasts longer than 7 days, the rate is classified as persistent atrial fibrillation. Permanent atrial fibrillation describes patients who have undergone failed cardioversions.

Classifications help to guide treatment options for patients. Based on the classification, patients might have rate or rhythm controlled by either medical or interventional therapies.[5]

Table 1 Atrial fibrillation classifications and definitions		
Classification	**Duration**	**Definition**
Paroxysmal Atrial Fibrillation	Within 7 d of onset	Episodes reverting to sinus rhythm spontaneously or with intervention Episodes can recur
Persistent Atrial Fibrillation	Greater than 7 d	Continuous atrial fibrillation
Long-standing Atrial Fibrillation	Greater than 12 mo	Continuous atrial fibrillation
Permanent Atrial Fibrillation		No further attempts made to restore sinus rhythm
Non-valvular Atrial Fibrillation		Atrial fibrillation with no evidence of mitral valve disease or intervention (rheumatic mitral stenosis, mitral valve repair or bioprosthetic valve)

Data from January CT, Wann LS, Alpert JS, et al. 2014 AHA/ACC/HRS guideline for the management of patients with atrial fibrillation: a report of the American College of Cardiology/American Heart Association Task Force on Practice Guidelines and the Heart Rhythm Society. J Am Coll Cardiol 2014;64(21):e1–76.

Pathophysiology

Structural heart diseases (hypertensive, valvular, and ischemic disease) account for most cases (85%) of permanent and persistent atrial fibrillation. Atrial fibrillation not caused by a structural heart problem accounts for only 15% of the total and is much less understood.[6]

Atrial fibrillation is thought to occur because of rapidly firing ectopic foci usually located in muscular sleeves of the proximal portion of the pulmonary veins.[7] Additionally, structurally related abnormal atrial tissue helps facilitate the perpetuation of atrial fibrillation.[8,9]

Patients suffering from recurrent episodes of atrial fibrillation are likely to have permanent atrial fibrillation, which provides evidence of heart remodeling. The likelihood of restoring sinus rhythm after cardioversion on those with persistent atrial fibrillation depends on the duration of the antecedent episode. Although reverse remodeling is possible, it is less likely to occur in patients with longstanding atrial fibrillation, thus reducing the success rate of cardioversion.[10]

Treatment

Treatment goals are based on the classification of atrial fibrillation. Short episodes of atrial fibrillation are more amenable to rhythm control, whereas in persistent atrial fibrillation, the focus becomes ventricular rate control. Regardless of the pattern of atrial fibrillation, patients will require some form of anticoagulation based on risk of thromboembolism.[11]

Restoration of sinus rhythm will improve patients' clinical symptoms, reduce likelihood of thromboembolism, and, in theory, reverse atrial remodeling. As previously mentioned, successful rhythm restoration is more likely with a shorter duration of atrial fibrillation. Guidelines recommend either electrical or pharmacologic cardioversion within the first 48 hours of onset. Patients do not require anticoagulation if cardioversion is done within 48 hours of onset, as risk of thromboembolism is much lower than in patients undergoing cardioversion later than that time period. Patients with a history of atrial fibrillation greater than 48 hours, or an unclear onset of when the arrhythmia started, will require 3 weeks of anticoagulation before cardioversion. If the patient has incomplete anticoagulation therapy, or if the patient is unstable and requires more urgent therapy, an alternative approach is available.

A *transesophageal* echocardiography (TEE) is an examination used to rule out any evidence of atrial thrombus before cardioversion. TEE is the most sensitive and specific technique to rule out any evidence of atrial thrombus (**Table 4** shows contraindications to TEE).[12] TEE can identify low velocity atrial blood flow, which places the patient at a higher risk for thrombus formation. Anticoagulation is continued for a month after successful cardioversion since atrial function does not immediately return.

Cardioversion

Direct current cardioversion is recommended for patients in atrial fibrillation or flutter in which rhythm control is desired. An external capacitor discharge type defibrillator delivers a coordinated shock. The shock delivered is coordinated with the QRS complex to avoid discharge during the repolarization phase or the T wave to prevent ventricular fibrillation. Normally, the sinoatrial node generates an impulse that transmits throughout the heart to induce myocardial depolarization. If enough external energy is delivered to heart, it will respond in a similar fashion as it does to an internal impulse, causing widespread depolarization and contraction. Immediately after the contraction is the recovery phase of the cardiac cycle, when the intrinsic pacemaker of the heart will attempt to regain control at this point.

Typically, 25 to 100 J are required for successful conversion of atrial fibrillation or flutter. Less energy is required when compared with delivering a shock for ventricular tachycardia, usually beginning at 200 J. Atrial fibrillation and flutter are abnormal rhythms contained within in the atria itself, which is in contrast to ventricular tachycardia, in which more myocardium requires electrical reset. The defibrillator may be set to deliver a set charge, such as 100 J, but the actual charge delivered to the myocardium may be different. The actual energy delivered by the defibrillator to the myocardium depends on multiple factors. The thoracic impedance is estimated to be about 50 Ω. Actual impedance varies depending on interelectrode distance, electrochest medium, the number of previous shocks, skin resistance, and the phase of ventilation during shock delivery. To help optimize delivery of energy, correct positioning of electro-pads is important. Ideally, an anteroposterior or anterolateral position is preferred. It is best to avoid placement of the electrodes directly over the sternum, as bone is a poor conductor of energy. Contraindications for cardioversion include known atrial thrombus, digitalis toxicity, sinus tachycardia, and multifocal tachycardia.[5]

A preprocedure evaluation must be completed for every patient similar to a presurgical evaluation. Furthermore, because electrical cardioversions are routinely performed out of the operating room, the additional items usually seen as a part of a routine NORA (Non Operating Room Anesthesia) safety checklist should be considered.

A complete history and physical examination should be obtained to develop an anesthetic plan for the procedure (**Box 1**).

A complete review of the patient's history and objective laboratory data are necessary to appropriately assess risk and appropriately develop an anesthetic plan to treat the patient. In rare situations, if objective cardiac function data are unavailable, then functional capacity by history can be used as a tool to grossly estimate the patient's cardiac status. Patient history should specifically include evaluation for obstructive sleep apnea using the STOP-BANG survey (**Table 2**).[13] In this survey, one point is given for each item that is present in the patient. If the patient scores ≥3, then they are considered to be at intermediate risk for obstructive sleep apnea. Additional precaution must be taken with these patients, as they will have a greater tendency to

---

Box 1
Preprocedure evaluation

Patient History

1. Patient identity and procedure confirmation

2. Medical History—focus on cardiac history, that is, history of heart attacks, strokes, previous cardioversions, cardiac stents, history of surgery (noting any history of endotracheal tube procedures)

3. Medication/Allergies—specifically noting last dose of any anticoagulant and antiarrhythmic medication

4. NPO status

5. Anesthesia history

6. Physical examination—airway evaluation, vital signs

7. Objective data—laboratory values (international normalized ratio), chest radiograph, electrocardiogram, echocardiogram

Table 2	
STOP-BANG assessment for obstructive sleep apnea	
S	Snoring loudly
T	Daytime tiredness
O	Observed apnea during sleep
P	High blood pressure
B	Body mass index >35 kg/m^2
A	Age 50 y
N	Neck circumference >40 cm
G	Male

Data from Chung F, Yegneswaran B, Liao P, et al. STOP questionnaire: a tool to screen patients for obstructive sleep apnea. Anesthesiology 2008;108(5):812–21.

obstruct during monitored anesthesia care. Oral airway or well-lubricated nasal trumpets should be available (nasal trumpets should be used with caution, as patients tend to be anticoagulated) if needed.

All objective studies should be reviewed carefully. Renal and hepatic laboratory results help determine the patient's ability to metabolize and eliminate anesthetic medications. Coagulation is status based usually on international normalized ratio or partial thromboplastin time, depending on which anticoagulant is used, and helps to determine the likelihood of clot development in the left atrial appendage. If the patient is in the subtherapeutic range or has missed recent doses of anticoagulant therapy, a TEE is indicated to assess for clot before cardioversion. A recent echocardiogram provides useful information on how the heart will react to a myocardial depressant. If the left and right ventricles seem normal with no serious valvular condition, the patient is considered to be at lower risk for an adverse cardiac-related complication.

Although there are no randomized, control trials regarding cardioversion and pregnancy, it is generally assumed to be safe for both mother and fetus. Electrical cardioversion is a rarely applied but highly effective tool in the treatment of maternal cardiac arrhythmias. Special attention should be given to choice of medications selected, and their ability to cross the placenta. Once fetal viability is reached, fetal heart rate monitoring is advised during cardioversion, and, if necessary, facilities for immediate cesarean section should be available.[14]

Intraoperative

Before patient arrival to the procedure room, the following items must be immediately available in case of an emergency, as most of these procedures are usually performed in a non–operating room setting (**Box 2**).

Before the procedure, the following standard monitors should be placed onto the patient: electrocardiogram, pulse oximeter, blood pressure cuff (opposite the

Box 2
Checklist items for out-of-operating room cardioversion
Airway equipment—laryngoscope, electrophysiology, nasal trumpet, oral airway, mask with bag valve mask
Suction
Intravenous access—should be checked before administration of sedation
Emergency medications—epinephrine, atropine, succinylcholine, and phenylephrine

extremity of where the intravenous line was placed) with automatic measurement set to every minute once induction of anesthesia begins. Additionally, continuous capnography should be available to all patients.[15] Although some propose administering atropine to help against vagotonic bradyarrhythmias after cardioversion, given the length of the procedure, it is uncommon to premedicate patients.[16]

When selecting an anesthetic agent, one must consider both the patient's comorbidities and type of procedure being done. An ideal agent would provide rapid hypnosis and rapid recovery and would not cause cardiac instability or induce nausea and vomiting, as this increases risk to patient and length of stay in the recovery area.

A combination of an opioid and fast-acting anxiolytic can be used to provide the adequate amnesia, sedation, and analgesia necessary for a cardioversion. The most common combination used is fentanyl and midazolam. Although this combination of medications provides all the necessary elements, including hemodynamic stability, required for a successful anesthetic for cardioversion, the dose is difficult to titrate. Midazolam causes minimal respiratory depression when used alone, but when administered with an opioid that has respiratory depressant effects, such as fentanyl, it acts in a synergistic manner to place the patient at an increased risk for apnea and hypoxemia, even after the procedure has ended.[17] Additionally, some studies suggest midazolam to be responsible for prolonged sedation well after the procedure.[18]

Alternatively, etomidate provides a hemodynamically stable anesthetic for those patients with cardiovascular compromise, such as reduced ejection fraction.[19] The use of etomidate results in minimal systemic vascular resistance changes and no myocardial depression. Patients with cardiovascular disease, especially those with reduced left ventricle ejection fraction, dependent on a higher perfusing pressure with a previous history of stroke, a history or previous myocardial infarction, or with severe aortic stenosis will benefit from maintaining a stable cardiac output during the procedure. An additional benefit with etomidate is that patients rarely have profound apnea, thereby minimizing the risk of assisted ventilation or even emergent tracheal intubation.[20] Etomidate is an excellent choice for cardioversion sedation, but it has some notable drawbacks to consider. Etomidate may activate seizure foci in some patients and at induction doses cause myocloniclike movements in approximately 50% of the patients. Etomidate has a high risk of causing postoperative nausea and vomiting, making it less ideal for scheduled outpatient cardioversions and TEEs.[21]

Pharmacologically, etomidate inhibits the enzyme 11-b-hydroxylase, which is a key component in production of cortisol from the adrenal gland. Enzyme deactivation may last up to 8 hours after a single induction dose of etomidate.[22]

Propofol is the most common induction/sedation medication in the operating room, intensive care unit, and emergency room. Propofol rapidly metabolizes in the liver and is renally excreted. Emergence occurs secondary to redistribution, with minimal residual sedative effects even with multiple repeated doses. Patients emerging from propofol do not experience a hangoverlike sensation. Additionally, propofol serves as an antiemetic and amnestic agent.[23] These properties make it an obvious choice for quick procedures such as cardioversions and TEEs, especially for those patients who are expected to return home after the procedure.[24]

Propofol does have profound myocardial depressant properties and reduces mean arterial pressure, more so than the other agents previously mentioned. Propofol vasodilates both the arterial and venous vasculature, thereby decreasing both preload and afterload. Propofol may cause apnea at induction doses. Propofol also causes a dose-dependent decrease in minute ventilation when used for sedation.

Postcardioversion

As mentioned, cardioversion is a short, painful procedure. The goal of the anesthetic is to provide adequate sedation with rapid recovery. Sedation may be prolonged if multiple attempts at cardioversion are necessary, but generally, the sedation lasts only several minutes.

After cardioversion, a decreased heart rate is often observed because of interruption in reentry circuits after depolarization of a critical mass of myocardium thus regaining sinus rhythm.[25] Systolic blood pressure may decrease because of decreased cardiac output from the slower heart rate. The amount of sedatives typically given does not usually result in clinically significant vasodilatation, unless agents are combined. Elderly patients with multiple comorbidities are more prone to profound hypotension when opioids are added.[26]

As the electrical connections of the heart are reset, there may be a period of hypotension that can be supported with low-dose vasopressors, such as phenylephrine. If the patient experiences significant bradycardia that is unstable, low-dose vagolytics or inotropic agents may be administered. Patients with intrinsic pacemakers should be monitored by the electrophysiology team, and normal sinus rhythm will return or the intrinsic pacemaker may take over and pace the patient. Extrinsic pacing can also be achieved by using the previously placed pacemaker/defibrillator pads.

Complications

A major challenge for the anesthesiologist during a cardioversion is to provide adequate amnesia and analgesia but avoid hemodynamic and respiratory compromise. Inadequate sedation may result in aspiration of stomach contents or airway obstruction of breathing. This risk is even higher in patients who are obese, who have obstructive sleep apnea, or have known difficult airways. It is imperative that the anesthesia team have on hand the resources to manage the airway in case of an emergency.

Cardioversion can provoke a bradyarrhythmia or tachyarrhythmia that may cause hemodynamic compromise. With atrial tachycardias, it is critical to deliver the shock in a synchronized fashion to avoid the R-on-T phenomenon that would lead to ventricular fibrillation. Conversely, the sinus node may not work properly after cardioversion, and a slow, junctional rhythm can occur. A temporary pacemaker may be necessary to correct this problem.

Patients are often on anticoagulation therapy for tachyarrhythmias or other comorbidities to reduce the risk of thromboembolism. While obtaining a thorough history and physical examination, it is crucial to determine what anticoagulation regimen the patient is on and to review the appropriate laboratory results. Transesophageal echocardiography is the gold standard for locating a clot within the heart, particularly the left atrium and left atrial appendage. TEE should be performed before elective cardioversion if there is any suspicion of thromboembolism. Cardioversion can result either in a stroke caused by embolism of clot that is already present or a new clot that forms after the procedure. Clot formation is unlikely in patients who have had an arrhythmia for less than 24 to 48 hours, and the use of preprocedural anticoagulation greatly reduces this risk.

Heart tissue damage can occur after high-energy or repeated shocks. However, significant damage is rare, and there are generally no long-term sequelae.

Skin burn may also occur as a result of high-energy or repeated shocks. Premedication with ibuprofen or other nonsteroidal anti-inflammatory drug may reduce the severity of burn pain.

Recovery

Care of the patient recovering from deep sedation required for cardioversion should adhere to the American Society of Anesthesiologists (ASA) practice guidelines for sedation and analgesia.[27] Despite avoidance of long-acting sedatives, patients may continue to be at significant risk for complications after the procedure is completed. Decreased procedural stimulation combined with delayed drug absorption and elimination in patients with depressed cardiac function may contribute to residual sedation and cardiorespiratory depression during the recovery period.

Most cardioversion patients are outpatients, and once they leave the hospital it is likely there will be no medical monitoring. Continued observation and monitoring of level of consciousness, vital signs, and oxygenation should be recorded at regular intervals immediately after the procedure. A nurse or other trained medical professional should be immediately available to monitor the patient and treat complications. Predetermined discharge criteria should be designated to minimize the risk for central nervous system and cardiorespiratory depression after discharge (**Box 3**).

Emergency Cardioversion

Most elective cardioversions are performed to treat atrial fibrillation or flutter in patients who are hemodynamically stable. Emergent cardioversion is performed when the patient has a tachyarrhythmia that has been present for less than 24 hours, when there is a need to convert to sinus rhythm and pharmacologic methods have failed, or the when the patient shows signs of hemodynamic compromise, such as hypotension, chest pain, difficulty breathing, or loss of consciousness. Emergency cardioversions are typically done in the emergency department. However, situations also arise in the non–operating room setting where it is necessary to emergently perform cardioversion on a hemodynamically unstable patient, and here the anesthesia team is involved.

Contraindications to emergency cardioversion include no clear onset of palpations in the patient's history, previous paroxysms of tachyarrhythmias and not on

---

Box 3
American Society of Anesthesiologists practice guidelines for discharge criteria after sedation and analgesia

1. Patients should be alert and oriented; infants and patients whose mental status was initially abnormal should have returned to their baseline status. Practitioners and parents must be aware that pediatric patients are at risk for airway obstruction should the head fall forward while the child is secured in a car seat.

2. Vital signs should be stable and within acceptable limits.

3. Use of scoring systems may assist in documentation of fitness for discharge.

4. Sufficient time (up to 2 h) should have elapsed after last administration of reversal agents (if necessary) to ensure that patients do not become renarcotized after reversal effects have worn off.

5. Outpatients should be discharged in the presence of a responsible adult who will accompany the patient home and be able to report any postprocedure complications.

6. Outpatients and their escorts should be provided with written instructions regarding postprocedure diet, medications, activities, and a phone number to be called in case of emergency.

From American Society of Anesthesiologists Task Force on sedation and analgesia by non-anesthesiologists. Practice guidelines for sedation and analgesia by non-anesthesiologists. Anesthesiology 2002;96(4):1012; with permission.

anticoagulation, or known atrial thrombus. Risks of emergency cardioversion are those associated with sedation, pain, failure to convert, stroke, and bradycardia requiring treatment.

Emergent cardioversions should be treated similarly to any emergent procedure. A thorough history and physical examination should be obtained, if possible, with special attention to nothing-by-mouth (NPO) status. If NPO status is unknown, the patient should be treated as having a full stomach. It may be necessary to induce general anesthesia and secure the airway against regurgitation and aspiration of gastric contents by endotracheal intubation. Succinylcholine, although not contraindicated, may precipitate bradyarrhythmias and exacerbate hyperkalemia.[28] Unless the patient is unconscious or in hemodynamic compromise, informed consent should be obtained for the procedure.

Currently, little evidence exists to guide the decision of whether sedation or general anesthesia for an emergency cardioversion is preferred. Careful attention to history and physical examination is paramount and will ultimately guide the anesthesia provider as to the best, safest anesthetic treatment plan.

Advanced cardiovascular life support protocol should be reviewed to determine if the abnormal rhythm is one that is considered shockable and whether synchronized or unsynchronized cardioversion is required. Initiation of cardiopulmonary resuscitation should not be delayed in cases where indicated.

Anesthesia for Transesophageal Echocardiography

TEE is a unique, specific diagnostic tool used by properly trained physicians to direct patient care. Any physicians using TEE should be specifically credentialed by their institution. The indications for TEE are generally based on the patient's condition. TEE is useful in preoperative surgical planning. Select patients need echocardiography for underlying structural (congenital), functional (valvular disease, cardiomyopathy), or ischemic cardiovascular disease.[29] TEE is commonly used in the electrophysiology laboratory to assess clot burden in patients undergoing cardioversion or ablation procedures. See **Table 3** for general indications for TEE and **Table 4** for contraindications to TEE according to the American Society of Echocardiography.[30]

This article focusses on TEE in the awake/sedated patient with an unsecured airway. There are differences in management when compared with an intubated patient and an intraoperative patient. Most transesophageal echocardiographic procedures are performed when the patient is moderately sedated. Patients should be NPO to a minimum of 6 hours and restrain from all intake at least 3 hours before the procedure. Patients with delayed gastric emptying or other aspiration risks may need a longer period of fasting. However, if there is any doubt as to status of the patient's airway or gastric emptying, it is prudent to secure the airway with endotracheal intubation. Although there is little evidence to support use of agents such as metoclopramide, minimizing the risk for residual gastric contents and aspiration is of paramount importance.[31] Intravenous access should be placed in the left arm if the examination is for detection of intracardiac shunts.

Standard monitors should be placed as per ASA guidelines for moderate sedation. End tidal capnography is strongly encouraged in these situations and mandated for deep sedation and general anesthesia. Careful assessment of the airway should be performed before the procedure, and proper equipment, including a functioning suction catheter, should be immediately available.

Awake patients usually have their oropharynx anesthetized topically to sedation, with viscous lidocaine, benzocaine, or Cetacaine as the most common agents used. Topical anesthesia can be achieved with spray, gargle, painting, or lozenge. All

Table 3
General indications for transesophageal echocardiography

General Indication	Specific Examples
1. Evaluation of cardiac and aortic structure and function in situations in which the findings will alter management and TTE is nondiagnostic or TTE is deferred because there is a high probability that it will be nondiagnostic	a. Detailed evaluation of the abnormalities in structures that are typically in the far field such as the aorta and the left atrial appendage b. Evaluation of prosthetic heart valves c. Evaluation of paravalvular abscesses (both native and prosthetic valves) d. Patients on ventilators e. Patients with chest wall injuries f. Patients with body habitus preventing adequate TTE imaging g. Patients unable to move into left lateral decubitus position
2. Intraoperative TEE	a. All open heart (ie, valvular) and thoracic aortic surgical procedures b. Use in some coronary artery bypass graft surgeries c. Noncardiac surgery when patients have known or suspected cardiovascular conditions that may impact outcomes
3. Guidance of transcatheter procedures	a. Guiding management of catheter-based intracardiac procedures (including septal defect closure or atrial appendage obliteration, and transcatheter valve procedures)
4. Critically ill patients	a. Patients in whom diagnostic information is not obtainable by TTE and this information is expected to alter management

From Hahn RT, Abraham T, Adams MS, et al. Guidelines for performing a comprehensive transesophageal echocardiographic examination: recommendations from the American Society of Echocardiography and the Society of Cardiovascular Anesthesiologists. J Am Soc Echocardiogr 2013;26(9):926; with permission.

methods used are equally effective, although patients preferred the spray technique.[32] Topical benzocaine carries the slight risk for methemoglobinemia. Supplemental oxygen and methylene blue should be readily available if that were to occur.

Commonly used sedative agents for TEE include benzodiazepines with midazolam. Many of these sedation drugs can be administered by a trained, supervised nurse under the guidelines of conscious sedation. However, if a patient has any indication for need of moderate to deep sedation, an anesthesia team should be involved. In patients who are robust and have relatively preserved cardiac function, propofol is the agent of choice. In compromised patients, etomidate may be used for hemodynamic preservation. Opioids are frequently administered as adjunct medications used to offset the discomfort of probe insertion and manipulation. Opioids have a synergistic effect when used with benzodiazepines. Intravenous reversal agents should be available to counter the effects of the benzodiazepines and opioids if necessary.

Once the patient's oropharynx has been topicalized with local anesthetic, the patient is placed in a left lateral decubitus position and a bite block is placed. Oxygen delivered via nasal cannula or modified nonrebreather is placed as sedation is administered. The probe is placed in the oropharynx and advanced when the patient

Table 4
List of absolute and relative contraindications for transesophageal echocardiography

Absolute Contraindications	Relative Contraindications
• Perforated viscus	• History of radiation to neck and mediastinum
• Esophageal stricture	• History of gastrointestinal surgery
• Esophageal tumor	• Recent upper gastrointestinal bleed
• Esophageal perforation, laceration	• Barrett's esophagus
• Esophageal diverticulum	• History of dysphagia
• Active upper gastrointestinal bleeding	• Restriction of neck mobility (severe cervical arthritis, atlantoaxial joint disease)
	• Symptomatic hiatal hernia
	• Esophageal varices
	• Coagulopathy, thrombocytopenia
	• Active esophagitis
	• Active peptic ulcer disease

From Hahn RT, Abraham T, Adams MS, et al. Guidelines for performing a comprehensive transeso-phageal echocardiographic examination: recommendations from the American society of echocardiography and the society of cardiovascular anesthesiologists. J Am Soc Echocardiogr 2013;26(9):927; with permission.

swallows. Communication between the anesthesia team and the echocardiography team will dictate length of sedation.

Once the TEE is completed, patients should be monitored in a postanesthesia care unit until they meet discharge criteria. The patient should also have nothing by mouth for more than an hour until all the local anesthetic and sedation medications have metabolized to decrease the risk of aspiration. Complications of cardioversion are relatively rare, with the most common issue being lip injury and hoarseness, and less commonly dental injury, minor pharyngeal bleeding, dysphagia, bronchospasm, laryngospasm, tracheal intubation, heart failure, and arrhythmia. Thankfully, esophageal perforation is an extremely rare event.

REFERENCES

1. Blomstrom-Lundqvist C, Scheinman M, Aliot E, et al. ACC/AHA/ESC guidelines for the management of patients with supraventricular arrhythmias–executive summary: a report of the American college of cardiology/American heart association task force on practice guidelines and the european society of cardiology committee for practice guidelines (writing committee to develop guidelines for the management of patients with supraventricular arrhythmias) developed in collaboration with NASPE-heart rhythm society. Circulation 2003;108:1871–909.
2. Saoudi N, Cosio F, Waldo A, et al. Classification of atrial flutter and regular atrial tachycardia according to electrophysiologic mechanism and anatomic bases: a statement from a joint expert group from the working group of arrhythmias of the european society of cardiology and the north american society of pacing and electrophysiology. J Cardiovasc Electrophysiol 2001;12:852.
3. Kalman J, Olgin JE, Saxon L, et al. Activation and entrainment mapping defines the tricuspid annulus as the anterior barrier in typical atrial flutter. Circulation 1996;94:398–406.
4. Markides V, Schilling RJ. Atrial fibrillation: classification, pathophysiology, mechanisms and drug treatment. Heart 2003;89(8):939–43.
5. Writing Committee Members, January CT, Wann LS, Alpert JS, et al. 2014 AHA/ACC/HRS guideline for the management of patients with atrial fibrillation: a report

of the American college of cardiology/American heart association task force on practice guidelines and the heart rhythm society. Circulation 2014;130(23): e199–267.

6. Chen Y, Xu S, Bendahhou S, et al. KCNQ1 gain-of-function mutation in familial atrial fibrillation. Science 2003;299:251–4.

7. Haïssaguerre M, Jaïs P, Shah D, et al. Spontaneous initiation of atrial fibrillation by ectopic beats originating in the pulmonary veins. N Engl J Med 1998;339:659–66.

8. Lau C, Tse H, Ayers G. Defibrillation-guided radiofrequency ablation of atrial fibrillation secondary to an atrial focus. J Am Coll Cardiol 1999;33:1217–26.

9. Allessie M, Lammers WJ, Smeets JR, et al. Total mapping of atrial excitation during acetylcholine-induced atrial flutter and fibrillation in the isolated canine heart. In: Kulbertus H, Olsson S, Schlepper M, editors. Atrial fibrillation. Molndal (Sweden): Lindgren and Soner; 1982. p. 44–62.

10. Tieleman R, Van Gelder I, Crijns H, et al. Early recurrences of atrial fibrillation after electrical cardioversion: a result of fibrillation-induced electrical remodeling of the atria? J Am Coll Cardiol 1998;31:167–73.

11. Albers G, Dalen J, Laupacis A, et al. Antithrombotic therapy in atrial fibrillation. Chest 2001;119:194S–206S.

12. Berger M, Schweitzer P. Timing of thromboembolic events after electrical cardioversion of atrial fibrillation or flutter: a retrospective analysis. Am J Cardiol 1998; 82:1545–7.

13. Chung F, Yegneswaran B, Liao P, et al. STOP questionnaire: a tool to screen patients for obstructive sleep apnea. Anesthesiology 2008;108:812–21.

14. Tromp CH, Nanne AC, Pernet PJ, et al. Electrical cardioversion during pregnancy: safe or not? Neth Heart J 2011;19(3):134–6.

15. American Society of Anesthesiologists. Standards for basic anesthestic monitoring. approved by the ASA house of delegates on October 21, 1986, last amended on October 20, 2010, and last affirmed on October 28, 2015.

16. Orko R. Anaesthesia for cardioversion: thiopentone with and without atropine premedication. Br J Anesth 1974;46:947–52.

17. Bailey P, Pace N, Ashburn M, et al. Frequent hypoxemia and apnea after sedation with midazolam and fentanyl. Anesthesiology 1990;73(5):826–30.

18. Canessa R, Lema G, Urzúa J, et al. Anesthesia for elective cardioversion: a comparison of four anesthetic agents. J Cardiothorac Vasc Anesth 1991;5(6):566–8.

19. Kalogridaki M, Souvatzis X, Mavrakis HE, et al. Anaesthesia for cardioversion: a prospective randomised comparison of propofol and etomidate combined with fentanyl. Hellenic J Cardiol 2011;52(6):483–8.

20. Stoelting R, Miller R. Intravenous anesthetics. Basics of anesthesia. 5th edition. Philadelphia: Churchill Livingstone; 2007. p. 97–111.

21. Morgan G, Mikhail M, Murray M. Nonvolatile anesthetic agents. Clinical anesthesiology. 4th edition. New York: McGraw-Hill; 2006. p. 179–204.

22. Fragen R, Shanks C, Molteni A, et al. Effects of etomidate on hormonal responses to surgical stress. Anesthesiology 1984;61:652–6.

23. Celik M, Dostbil A, Aksoy M, et al. Is infusion of subhypnotic propofol as effective as dexamethasone in prevention of postoperative nausea and vomiting related to laparoscopic cholecystectomy? a randomized controlled trial. Biomed Res Int 2015;2015:349806.

24. Barash P, Cullen B, Stoelting R, et al. Intravenous anesthetics. Clinical anesthesia. 6th edition. Philadelphia: Lippincott and Williams & Wilkins; 2009. p. 444–63.

25. Zipes D, Fischer J, King R, et al. Termination of ventricular fibrillation in dogs by depolarizing a critical amount of myocardium. Am J Cardiol 1975;36:37–44.

26. Reeves J, Glass P, Lubersky D, et al. Intravenous anesthetics. In: Miller RD, editor. Miller's anaesthesia. 7th edition. Philadelphia: Churchill Livingstone Elsevier; 2010. p. 724–5, 748–749.

27. Gross J, Bailey P, Connis R, et al. Practice guidelines for sedation and analgesia by non-anesthesiologists: an updated report by the american society of anesthesiologists task force on sedation and analgesia by non-anesthesiologists. Anesthesiology 2002;96:1004–17.

28. Stoneham MD. Anesthesia for cardioversion. Anaesthesia 1996;51:565–70.

29. Writing Committee Members. Statement on transesophageal echocardiography. Committee of origin: economics. American Society of Anesthesiologists 2015;1–6.

30. Writing Committee Members. 2013 ASE Guidelines for performing a comprehensive trans esophageal echocardiographic examination: recommendations from the American society of echocardiography and society of cardiovascular anesthesiologists. J Am Soc Echocardiogr 2013;26:921–64.

31. American Society of Anesthesiologists Committee. Practice guidelines for preoperative fasting and the use of pharmacologic agents to reduce the risk of pulmonary aspiration: application to healthy patients undergoing elective procedures: an updated report by the american society of anesthesiologists committee on standards and practice parameters. Anesthesiology 2011;114:495–511.

32. Smith JL, Opekun A, Graham DY. Controlled comparison of topical an- esthetic agents in flexible upper gastrointestinal endoscopy. Gastrointest Endosc 1985; 31:255–8.

Anesthesia for Routine and Advanced Upper Gastrointestinal Endoscopic Procedures

Christopher D. Sharp, MD, MS[a], Ezekiel Tayler, DO[b],
Gregory G. Ginsberg, MD[c],*

KEYWORDS

- Anesthesia for endoscopy • Sedation for endoscopy
- Sedation for endoscopic retrograde cholangiopancreatography
- Anesthesia for per-oral endoscopic myotomy

KEY POINTS

- Endoscopic procedures have expanded in their intensity and complexity.
- Sedation for endoscopic procedures has evolved to support that increase in intensity and complexity.
- Enhanced anesthesia services emphasize safety and permit tolerance for patients undergoing complex endoscopic procedures.

INTRODUCTION

Diagnostic and therapeutic indications for gastrointestinal (GI) endoscopy have increased as technological advances continue to favor minimally invasive techniques. The role and level of involvement of the anesthesia team in the delivery of sedation in the endoscopy suite may vary according to need. Multiple professional associations have issued guidelines and recommendations on sedation and sedation levels to be delivered during outpatient endoscopic procedures. The American Society of Anesthesiologists (ASA) Task Force published guidelines for nonanesthesiologist-driven sedation and analgesia. The ASA House of Delegates on October 15, 2014 in fact released the following statement: "There is no circumstance when it is considered

Disclosure: Dr G.G. Ginsberg has nothing to disclose.

[a] University of Tennessee Health Science Center, Memphis, TN 38163, USA; [b] Cardiothoracic ICU, Lankenau Medical Center, 100 East Lancaster Avenue, 2nd Floor Heart Pavilion, Wynnewood, PA 19096, USA; [c] Gastroenterology Division, University of Pennsylvania, Perelman School of Medicine, Penn Medicine, Abramson Cancer Center, Perelman Center for Advanced Medicine, South Pavilion, 7th Floor, 3400 Civic Center Boulevard, Philadelphia, PA 19104, USA
* Corresponding author.
E-mail address: gregory.ginsberg@uphs.upenn.edu

acceptable for a person to experience emotional or psychological duress or untreated pain amenable to safe intervention while under a physician's care."

It is important to understand that in routine practice, procedures vary greatly between GI endoscopic facilities, and familiarity with one's institutional guidelines is necessary to ensure the safe and efficient care for patients and practitioners. However, it is safe to say that therapeutic endoscopic procedures (eg, polyp resections, endoscopic retrograde cholangiopancreatography [ERCP], dilation, and biopsies) are more likely to require anesthesia compared with routine screening procedures.

Requests for anesthesiology in the endoscopy suite often depend on the gastroenterologist's preference, patient population, and expected time of the procedure. The choice of anesthetic depends on patient comorbidities, duration, procedure, and the abilities of the gastroenterologist. Most routine procedures are performed on an outpatient basis with an expectation for a quick recovery. Routine screening in outpatient GI care may vary on a regional basis, but most patients are screened the day of procedure. Although most procedures are performed under sedation, the ability to control the airway and intubate a patient in an emergency is crucial. The presence of an endoscope impairs ready access to the airway, so careful planning and preparation before the procedure is important if intervention may be required.

There has been an increase in anesthesia involvement in endoscopic procedures since 2000, with 98% to 99% of endoscopies being done with sedation/general anesthesia.[1] Reasons for this increase include:

1. An increase in endoscopists who do not want to divide their attention between performing the procedure and maintaining the sedation
2. Endoscopy procedures are becoming more common in children, whose cooperation may be gained only with the administration of general anesthesia
3. Propofol offers faster and more complete patient recovery leading to greater endoscopist and patient satisfaction[2]

OPERATING ROOM COMMUNICATION

One of the crucial factors of the operating room environment that leads to overall safety of anesthesia is communication between all parties involved in the case. There is also a standardization of processes that have been well established that lead to a reliability built into the operating room environment. A common problem with anesthesia being delivered in remote (nonoperating room) locations is the absence of the standardization of communication and the process. This lack of communication and standardization potentially leads to:

- Decrease in efficiency in scheduling, resulting in inefficient patient preparation
- Equipment that is not maintained properly
- Greater variation in the physical set-up of the room, resulting in the decreased familiarity with the environment and equipment
- Delays in receiving needed patient information
- Inadequate monitoring for the case
- Nursing and support personnel who do not have the proper knowledge base in order to efficiently and safely take care of the patient
- Working with staff whom the anesthesiologist has not met or being unfamiliar with the staffs skill sets

The potential problems from the mentioned deficiencies are all magnified do to the distance that NORA locations are from the core operating room areas and subsequent help from colleagues.[3] Most of these can be addressed by allowing for an environment that encourages communication between all parties involved in the care of the patient and the implementation of a preinduction check list. This list should at a minimum verify the patient's name, surgery/procedure and site, surgeon, surgical instruments needed for the case, antibiotics needed, and any anesthetic concerns.

PHARMACOLOGIC STRATEGIES

There is no one size fits all cocktail for cases in the GI suite. The depth of the anesthetic will rely on several factors, including the patient comorbidities and type and duration of the procedure. Paralytic agents are rarely required in the GI suite except to intubate. Medications to facilitate monitored anesthesia care (MAC) or mild sedation are at the discretion of the anesthesia provider. Propofol, dexmedetomindine, ketamine, midazolam, and fentanyl are all medications that may be used in a GI suite. Titration of the medications to effect is an important task. An end tidal CO_2 monitor is valuable in monitoring the patient's ventilator status, and should be used to diagnose and treat airway obstruction, potential medication side effects, and cardiopulmonary depression.

The sedation process is an art as much as a science. Patient safety must be maintained while ensuring procedural comfort and providing the endoscopist with a suitable condition to work in. ASA standard monitoring is absolutely required, including the ability to monitor $ETCO_2$. Open and frequent communication with the proceduralist, including a preprocedural time-out, should occur regularly. The GI endoscopy suite is a high turnover area, and there is often pressure to move ahead at an accelerated pace, but this pressure should be resisted if patient care issues arise. The anesthesia team is there to ensure that the facility has the medication, equipment, facilities, and staff necessary to treat and reasonable contingency before it arises. In the gastrointestinal procedures section of this article, the authors put forth suggestions for the type of anesthetic to be delivered for specific procedures. It is important to note that although most patients may tolerate MAC for an EGD, not every patient's tolerance level is the same. Each patient and procedure should be analyzed and treated appropriately based on physician judgment and experience. To help with the decision of whether to protect the airway or not in the GI suite, the following algorithm in **Box 1** has been developed.

Any score of 4 or greater or any patient with full stomach or gastric outlet obstruction should warrant consideration of securing the airway. If GI status of the patient is not clear, then one should consult with the GI attending. There is no substitution, however, for the thoughtful evaluation and judgment of the anesthesia team.

NONPHARMACOLOGIC STRATEGIES

On rare occasions, some patients who may opt to not receive sedation for certain GI procedures. Routine esophagogastroduodenostomy (EGD) and colonoscopy are 2 examples in which sedation may not be necessary. The pain and discomfort for the EGD and colonoscopy generally occur during insertion of the scope and insufflation of the bowels. Visceral pain from insufflation can be severe but subjective from 1 patient to another. It is not the recommendation of the authors to pose the option for absence of analgesia and amnesia for GI procedures but merely for providers to be aware that such a route exists.

GASTROINTESTINAL PROCEDURES
Routine Esophagogastroduodenostomy

EGD, also known as an upper GI endoscopy (UGI), permits direct visualization of the esophagus, stomach, and duodenum. Common indications for diagnostic EGD

Box 1
Gastrointestinal suite intubation algorithm

1. Body Mass Index
   Less than 25 = 0
   25 to 35 = 1
   Greater than 35 = 2

2. Status of procedure and Time of Day Done
   Elective/urgent = 0
   Emergent due to Upper GI bleeding = 4
   Emergent due to Lower GI Bleeding = 2
   Start time after 1800 = 1

3. Gastrointestinal Status
   NPO = 0
   No/controlled gastroesophageal reflux disease (GERD) = 0
   Active GERD = 1
   History of aspiration = 1
   NG tube in place = 1

4. Pulmonary/Hemodynamic/Cardiac Status
   Stable = 1
   Unstable = 2
   Pulmonary hypertension = 1
   Requires supplemental oxygen = 1

5. Airway
   Mallampati score less than or equal to 2 = 0
   Mallampatis score greater than 3 = 1
   Confirmed or suspected OSA = 1

---

include the evaluation of dysphagia and odynophagia, reflux or heartburn symptoms, abdominal pain and dyspepsia, unexplained nausea, vomiting, weight loss, and anemia.[4] Diagnostic EGD is routinely performed as an outpatient procedure with sedation with analgesia or MAC with propofol sedation.[5] Simple diagnostic EGD with forceps tissue biopsy is a relatively quick procedure, with scope-in time generally under 15 to 30 minutes. Consideration pertaining to airway protection and intubation of the trachea should be entertained in circumstances with patients who may have retained gastric or esophageal contents, patients with motility disorders, or patients with mechanical or gastric outlet obstruction.

Advanced Upper Gastrointestinal Procedures

An upper GI endoscopy procedure may be either a diagnostic or therapeutic procedure. Esophageal and anastomotic strictures are treated with dilation using tapper-tip catheters advanced over a guide wire, or under direct endoscopic visualization with through-the-scope balloon inflation. Esophageal stents may be routinely placed for palliation of malignant dysphagia under endoscopic with or without fluoroscopic guidance. These procedures are typically performed under sedation with analgesia, or under MAC with propofol sedation.[6]

Patients with compromised respiratory status, proximal esophageal malignancies, and known (or suspected) esophagotracheal fistula may be considered for endotracheal intubation. Enteral stenting is effective in palliating malignant gastric outlet obstruction. If retained gastric contents are known or suspected, endotracheal intubation is advised to prevent aspiration.

Percutaneous endoscopic gastrostomy (PEG) is among the most widely performed therapeutic endoscopic procedures. Unlike most EGD procedures in which the patient is in the left lateral decubitus position, PEG is performed with the patient supine. Procedural stimulation is highest during PEG insertion during the transcutaneous needle insertion and when the gastrostomy tube is pulled though the gastric and anterior abdominal walls.[7]

Acute upper GI bleed is another common indication for urgent endoscopy. Endoscopic hemostatic therapy has been demonstrated to improve patient outcomes. The type of sedation and need for airway protection should be individualized for each case. UGI bleeding may be categorized on the basis of a known or suspected source of the bleed: variceal or nonvariceal. Endotracheal intubation should be considered in patients with suspected retained blood in the stomach or esophagus. Patients with variceal bleeding typically have advanced liver disease, thrombocytopenia, coagulopathy, and portal hypertension. Patients with variceal bleeding are at particularly high risk for adverse events including aspiration of blood. In many liver patients, an accompanying history of substance or ethanol abuse may make these cases particularly challenging.

Epithelial-based neoplasms are now routinely treated using endoscopic mucosal resection (EMR) techniques. EMR techniques may employ special accessories attached to the distal aspect of the endoscope. When the gastroscope is inserted, hyperextension of the neck may be requested to allow passage of the scope though the laryngopharynx. EMR procedures typically take considerably longer (30–60 minutes). EMR procedures require a degree of precision to perform, and a quiet field is necessary for the proceduralist to be successful. Often, this technique requires that the patient be heavily sedated to reduce the chance of movement. Postresection bleeding is an anticipated potential adverse event, and the team should be alert should the need to perform endoscopic measures to achieve immediate hemostasis. EMR specimen retrieval should be undertaken with secure devices to mitigate the risk of accidental dislodgement of the specimen during withdrawal of the specimen in the esophagus or upper airway.

Endoscopic submucosal dissection (ESD) is an advanced form of EMR that employs oncological microdissection techniques to resect and retrieve larger lesions in an en bloc fashion. These techniques, pioneered in Japan, are being gradually adopted at specialty centers around the globe. These procedures require more time, and general anesthesia with endotracheal intubation is the norm.[8] In cases expected to extend beyond 1 hour, intermittent compression stocking should be used for thromboembolism prophylaxis.

Barrett esophagus Is a common condition in which the distal portion of the esophagus undergoes change at a cellular level that may be recognized on endoscopy. Patients with this condition have an increased risk for developing esophageal adenocarcinoma. Patients with high-risk features of Barrett esophagus may be offered endoscopic eradication therapy employing EMR and/or mucosal ablation techniques. Radiofrequency ablation (RFA) has become the standard technique for treatment of Barrett esophagus. Barrett RFA is routinely performed as an outpatient procedure. RFA catheters are advanced over an endoscopically placed guide wire, or affixed to the tip of the endoscope, and ablation is performed under endoscopic visualization. These procedures typically are of longer duration (30–40 minutes) and require multiple reinsertions of the endoscope. Patients may experience pain or discomfort during the actual ablation maneuver. For these procedures, MAC with propofol sedation is typically preferred.

Balloon-Assisted Deep Enteroscopy

Balloon-assisted deep enteroscopy (BADENT) employs dedicated systems with very long endoscopes and a sliding overtube with balloons distally. As the proceduralist advances the enteroscope and overtube assembly, the balloon(s) are intermittently inflated and the small intestine reduced to allow for incremental insertion of the endoscope deep within the small intestine. BADENT is used to evaluate patients with obscure GI bleeding and abnormalities seen on radiographic or capsule endoscopy studies. BADENT procedures are useful in patients with surgically altered anatomy, such as after roux-n- y gastric bypass. These procedures are longer in duration and associated with considerable inter-procedural discomfort. BADENT procedures are typically performed under MAC with propofol sedation.[9]

Endoscopic Ultrasound

Endoscopic ultrasound (EUS) employs a modified endoscope with a high-frequency ultrasound transducer at the tip. Placement of the EUS probe into close proximity to the organ of interest allows high-resolution imaging. EUS is used to evaluate both mural lesions of the upper digestive tract and extramural structures adjacent to the UGI tract. EUS is useful for ultrasound characterization and EUS-guided fine needle aspiration (FNA) of lesions within the UGI tract wall, mediastinal structures, pancreas, and surrounding peritoneal structures. EUS and EUS-FNA have become routine outpatient procedures. EUS scopes have a larger outside diameter and a longer fixed length at the instrument tip compared with the standard EGD scope. EUS and EUS-FNA may require higher levels of sedation compared with standard diagnostic EGD procedures.[10]

Endoscopic Retrograde Cholangiopancreatography

ERCP combines endoscopic and fluoroscopic techniques to obtain radiographic imaging of the pancreatic and biliary systems. The ERCP scope, which is modified with side-viewing optics and is equipped with an elevator lever to direct catheters passed thought the accessory channel, is advanced to the second portion of the duodenum to localize the ampulla of Vater. ERCP is used principally for therapeutic purposes. The most common indications for ERCP are choledocolithiasis, palliation of malignant biliary obstruction, bile leak and evaluation, and management of benign biliary strictures.

ERCP presents multiple challenges to the endoscopist and anesthesia team. The procedure is performed in a room with dedicated fluoroscopy equipment. This can constrain the room for anesthesia personnel and equipment. Second, the room is typically darkened to enhance fluoroscopic image interpretation. Third, ERCP is conventionally performed with the patient in a modified prone position to optimize cholangiography and pancreatography, although ERCP may well be performed with the patient supine. Fourth, these are high-intensity procedures of longer duration (60–90 minutes). Finally, these patients are often acutely or chronically ill, hospitalized, and may have had recent abdominal surgery.

MAC anesthesia with propofol sedation for ERCP has improved the experience of patient, endoscopist, and staff. However, in some circumstances, the patient and proceduralist may be better served with GA and endotracheal intubation. Each patient's case should be individually considered by the anesthesia team, and a determination as to the optimal approach be arrived at collaboratively among the endoscopist, nursing, and anesthesia.[11] The authors developed a scoring system used to consider elective ETI for in patients undergoing ERCP. This system takes into consideration the patient's body mass index (BMI), aspiration risk, hemodynamics, airway, and intangibles like evening or weekend case. It provides a guide to more objectively settle on a plan.

Patients who have recently undergone abdominal surgeries (eg, postliver transplant stricture, postlaparoscopic cholecystectomy bile leak, post-trauma pancreatic leak) are ill-suited for the prone position and must be done supine. This positioning is better supported with GA and ETI.

Natural Orifice Transluminal Endoscopic Surgery

Natural orifice transluminal endoscopic surgery (NOTES) is a concept born of minimally invasive surgery and endoscopy. NOTES procedures are intended to address conditions that historically had been accessed with iatrogenic abdominal, pelvic, or thoracic incisions. The NOTES concept allows entry into the mediastinal or peritoneal space through a natural orifice (eg, mouth, anus, or vagina). Theoretically, there are many possible applications for NOTES. Two have become sufficiently established for discussion here.

Endoscopic cystgastrostomy

Endoscopic cystgastrostomy has become first-line therapy for the +patient with symptomatic pancreatic pseudocysts and infected pancreatic walled-off necrosis.[12] These procedures are typically conducted in the ERCP procedure room employing EUS imaging and fluoroscopy. The EUS scope is advanced into the stomach or duodenum, and the pseudocyst cavity is identified. A needle is passed under EUS and fluoroscopic guidance into the pseudocyst cavity. A guide wire is advanced thought the needle and coiled in the pseudocyst cavity. After the tract between the gastric and pseudocyst wall is dilated with a balloon catheter, at least 1 plastic stent is placed to create a durable cystgastrostomy. Recently, this NOTES device has been adapted to simplify the process with an EUS-guided thermal tip catheter that allows tunneling directly into the pseudocyst cavity. Once inside the pseudocyst, a large-diameter fully covered metal mesh stent is deployed. In NOTES procedures, technical proficiency is a must. Patients must be well sedated to permit the procedure to proceed uninterrupted.

The optimal patient position for endoscopic cystgastrostomy has not been established and may be performed prone, supine, or in the left-lateral decubitus position. The patient's general medical condition is taken into consideration to determine the means of sedation. Patients with septic physiology should be managed with GA and ETI. However, patients with sterile fluid collections and robust hemodynamics are well managed with MAC using propofol sedation. Once the communication into the pseudocyst is created, the cyst contents drain readily into the stomach. Measures to prevent aspiration must be employed. The gastric contents are vigorously aspirated with the endoscope, and may be aided by placing the patient in reverse Trendelenburg position.

Per-Oral Endoscopic Myotomy

Achalasia is a disease of esophageal dysmotility. Achalasia patients lose peristalsis, and the lower-esophageal sphincter (LES) fails to properly relax. Patients with achalasia may experience dysphagia, retained contents in the esophagus, esophageal dilation, and regurgitation of ingested contents. The per-oral endoscopic myotomy (POEM) procedure is intended to replicate the operative Heller myotomy. As the name implies, the POEM procedure is performed endoscopically, without an abdominal or thoracic incision. A submucosal injection of saline is made in the midesophagus. This creates a space within the submucosal layer. An incision is made though the mucosal to permit the endoscope to enter the submucosal space. Alternating injection and spray coagulation are used to create a submucosal tunnel to and several centimeters beyond the LES. Using specially designed tools developed initially for ESD, the exposed circular muscle layer is cut to create a long myotomy in the distal esophagus, through the LES, and into the gastric cardia. Once the myotomy has been completed, the endoscope is withdrawn from the tunnel, and the entry site is closed with clips. POEM is most commonly performed in an operating room setting, as well as properly equipped high-intensity endoscopy units. The procedure is performed in the supine position and with GA and ETI.[13]

Although POEM patients are instructed to limit their diet to clear liquids only for 2 days prior to the procedure and have fasted a minimum of 6 hours prior to the procedure, many achalasia patients will still retain some gastric contents in the esophagus. Reverse Trendelenburg position and rapid induction sequence are recommended to reduce the risk of aspiration during intubation. Compression stockings are used for deep vein thrombosis prophylaxis. The POEM procedure is performed with CO_2 as the insufflation gas; the abdomen is periodically palpated to assess for tension capnoperitoneum. If this occurs, an angiocatheter may be inserted for decompression if necessary. Airway pressure is monitored for capnothorax. Up to 30% of patients will have chest discomfort immediately on awakening. Although this rapidly dissipates in most patients, narcotic analgesia may be used for pain management. Agents that may interfere with clotting (eg, ketorolac) should be avoided.

SUMMARY

UGI endoscopic procedures range from simple diagnostic procedures to complex advanced, minimally invasive surgeries. Advances in therapeutic endoscopy have relied on safe and effective anesthesia support. The level of anesthesia and airway management varies with the type of the procedure and the patient condition. Endoscopists, nurses, and anesthesia providers must work in a collaborative and coordinated way to optimize patient outcomes.

REFERENCES

1. De Villers WJS. Anesthesiology and gastroenterology. Anesthesiol Clin 2009;27: 57–70.
2. Goulson DT, Fragneto RY. Anesthesia for gastrointestinal endoscopic procedures. Anesthesiol Clin 2009;27:71–85.
3. Frankel A. Patient safety: anesthesia in remote locations. Anesthesiol Clin 2009; 27:127–39.
4. ASGE Standards of Practice Committee, Early DS, Ben-Menachem T, Decker GA, et al. Appropriate use of GI endoscopy. Gastrointest Endosc 2012;75:1127–31.
5. Cohen LB, Wecsler JS, Gaetano JN, et al. Endoscopic sedation in the United States: results from a nationwide survey. Am J Gastroenterol 2006;101:967–74.
6. Levitzky BE, Lopez R, Dumot JA, et al. Moderate sedation for elective upper endoscopy with balanced propofol versus fentanyl and midazolam alone: a randomized clinical trial. Endoscopy 2012;44(01):13–20.
7. Horiuchi A, Nakayama Y, Kajiyama M, et al. Effectiveness of outpatient percutaneous endoscopic gastrostomy replacement using esophagogastroduodenoscopy and propofol sedation. World J Gastrointest Endosc 2012;4(2):45–9.
8. Nonaka T, Inamori M, Miyashita T, et al. Feasibility of deep sedation with a combination of propofol and dexmedetomidine hydrochloride for esophageal endoscopic submucosal dissection. Dig Endosc 2016;28(2):145–51.

9. Sethi S, Thaker AM, Cohen J, et al. Monitored anesthesia care without endotracheal intubation is safe and efficacious for single-balloon enteroscopy. Dig Dis Sci 2014;59(9):2184–90.

10. Cases Viedma E, Andreo García F, Flandes Aldeyturriaga J, et al. Tolerance and safety of 5 models of sedation during endobronchial ultrasound. Arch Bronconeumol 2016;52(1):5–11.

11. Buxbaum J, Roth N, Motamedi N, et al. Anesthetist -directed sedation favors success of advanced endoscopic procedures. Am J Gastroenterol 2017;112(2): 290–6.

12. Fabbri C, Luigiano C, Maimone A, et al. Endoscopic ultrasound-guided drainage of pancreatic fluid collections. World J Gastrointest Endosc 2012;4(11):479–88.

13. Yang D, Pannu D, Zhang Q, et al. Evaluation of anesthesia management, feasibility and efficacy of peroral endoscopic myotomy (POEM) for achalasia performed in the endoscopy unit. Endosc Int Open 2015;3(4):E289–95.

Anesthesia for Colonoscopy and Lower Endoscopic Procedures

John Michael Trummel, MD, MPH[a],*, Vinay Chandrasekhara, MD[b],
Michael L. Kochman, MD[b]

KEYWORDS

- Anesthesia • Colonoscopy • Deep sedation • Lower endoscopic procedures
- Moderate sedation • Outcomes • Propofol

KEY POINTS

- Demand for anesthesiologist-assisted sedation is expanding for gastrointestinal lower endoscopic procedures and may add to the cost of these procedures.
- The vast majority of lower endoscopy can be accomplished with either no, moderate, or deep sedation; general anesthesia and active airway management are rarely needed.
- Propofol-based sedation has advantages in terms of satisfaction and recovery over other modalities, but moderate sedation using benzodiazepines and opiates work well for low-risk patients and procedures.
- No sedation for routine colonoscopy works well for selected patients and eliminates sedation related risks.
- There is no difference in outcome measures based on sedation received.

INTRODUCTION

In developed countries, most lower endoscopic procedures receive some type of sedation/anesthesia. Sedation is typically utilized for several congruent reasons: patients want a favorable experience; endoscopists want reasonable technical conditions, and both want optimal patient safety and procedural outcomes. Sedation can be administered by the endoscopy team or by an anesthesia specialist. However, adding anesthesia services may add significantly to the cost of these procedures; this concern needs to be considered when planning an optimal sedation strategy. The purpose of this article is to review relevant recent literature surrounding sedation practice for colonoscopy and lower endoscopic procedures. Specific considerations

[a] Anesthesiology, Dartmouth Hitchcock Medical Center, 1 Medical Center Drive, Lebanon, NH 03756, USA; [b] Gastroenterology Division, Perelman School of Medicine at the University of Pennsylvania, 3400 Civic Center Boulevard, Philadelphia, PA 19104, USA
* Corresponding author.
E-mail address: John.M.Trummel@hitchcock.org

Anesthesiology Clin 35 (2017) 679–686
http://dx.doi.org/10.1016/j.anclin.2017.08.007
1932-2275/17/© 2017 Elsevier Inc. All rights reserved.

include a review of best sedation practice, safety, quality, and outcomes related to sedation, and the cost profile of differing regimens.

SEDATION PRACTICE FOR LOWER ENDOSCOPY

Anesthesiologists define sedation on a continuum from mild sedation to general anesthesia (**Table 1**).[1] Lower endoscopy can be performed anywhere on this spectrum. Traditionally, most routine lower endoscopy has been performed in the United States with endoscopist-supervised moderate sedation using a benzodiazepine and opiate combination. More recently, deep sedation with propofol administered by an anesthesia provider has increased in utilization. Occasional patients, usually because of personal preference, may choose not to have any sedation for colonoscopy. Although most standard lower endoscopic procedures can be performed with minimal or moderate sedation, complex interventional lower endoscopic procedures or those that are longer in duration may require deeper levels of sedation (**Box 1**). Rarely, specific patients may require general anesthesia with active airway management.

Although most patients now receive sedation or anesthesia for lower endoscopy, several studies have evaluated the no sedation option to determine procedural effectiveness and/or quality. A 1999 study randomized 70 self-selected patients to either moderate sedation or sedation as needed. In the sedation as needed group, 94% had the procedure completed without any sedation. Most (91%) were very satisfied, and the remainder were somewhat satisfied with the overall experience. All of the patients in the moderate sedation arm were very satisfied with their care. In the sedation as needed group, there were fewer episodes of hypotension and hypoxemia and lower overall charges. The authors concluded that a sedation as needed approach is viable for selected patients.[2] More recently, a community-based endoscopy center trialed a patient-selected option for sedation as needed for outpatient colonoscopy and reported that over a 6-month period 27.6% of patients selected this option. Over 80% of the patients completed the examination without sedation, and of these, 97.4% were satisfied with their comfort during the procedure. The authors concluded that offering unsedated colonoscopy with sedation as needed is effective and feasible in a typical US population.[3] The advantage to no sedation is avoidance of sedation-related complications and minimal post-procedural recovery as well as potentially decreased cost and increased efficiency.

Historically, most patients have received endoscopist-directed moderate sedation. However, a recent study using a combination of Medicare and commercial billing data to assess utilization of anesthesia services in gastrointestinal (GI) endoscopy found a steadily increasing trend in the use of such services. The use of anesthesia increased from around one-third of all patients in 2009 to about one-half of all patients in 2013, and most were considered low-risk patients (defined by American Society of Anesthesiologists [ASA] patient classification 1 and 2).[4] The authors characterized anesthesia care for ASA class 1 and 2 patients as discretionary care, but did note for this analysis that the ASA class was unavailable and had to be modeled. They were also unable to differentiate between simple and complex procedures. Even so, it appears most anesthesia services are used in discretionary cases, and the authors estimate this may cost upwards of $1.5 billion annually in the United States.

The main driver of this shift in sedation care is due to the use of propofol deep sedation. Although other agents have been used for sedation for colonoscopy, none have proven to be equal or superior to propofol in various domains. These advantages include rapid-onset and recovery with minimal postprocedural adverse effects, profound procedural amnesia, good procedural operating conditions, and excellent patient and provider satisfaction.[5] The main alternative to propofol is moderate sedation with a combination

Table 1
American Society of Anesthesiologists sedation continuum

Level of Sedation	Responsiveness	Airway	Spontaneous Ventilation	Cardiovascular Function
Minimal	Normal to verbal stimulation	Unaffected	Unaffected	Unaffected
Moderate	Purposeful response to verbal or tactile stimulation	No intervention required	Adequate	Usually maintained
Deep	Purposeful response after repeated or painful stimulation	Intervention may be required	May be inadequate	Usually maintained
General anesthesia	Unarousable even with painful stimulation	Intervention often required	Frequently inadequate	May be impaired

Adapted from American Society of Anesthesiologists. Continuum of depth of sedation: definition of general anesthesia and levels of sedation/analgesia. Available at: www.asahq.org/~/media/Sites/ASAHQ/Files/Public/Resources/standards-guidelines/continuum-of-depth-of-sedation-definition-of-general-anesthesia-and-levels-of-sedation-analgesia.pdf. Accessed August 10, 2017; with permission.

Box 1
Lower endoscopic procedures

1. Standard lower endoscopic procedures
   a. Elective colonoscopy
   b. Elective sigmoidoscopy
   c. Diagnostic lower endoscopic ultrasound

2. Interventional lower endoscopic procedures
   a. Urgent colonoscopy (eg, acute lower GI bleed)
   b. Endoscopic mucosal resection
   c. Endoscopic submucosal dissection
   d. Stricture management (dilation or endoprosthetic placement)
   e. Fistula/perforation management
   f. Lower endoscopic ultrasound with fine needle aspiration
   g. Natural orifice transluminal endoscopic surgery

---

of a benzodiazepine and opiate. Although these agents work well for most patients, some will have procedural recall, poor intraprocedural sedation, prolonged recovery, and postprocedural emesis. A study in 2005 evaluated the actual depth of sedation in patients having different endoscopic procedures even though the targeted sedation level was moderate. The study found that for colonoscopy, 11% percent of patients were at a deep sedation level at every sedation assessment, and 45% had deep sedation at least once.[6] This confirms the experience of most endoscopists who realize that although a benzodiazepine and opiate combination targeting moderate sedation works well for most patients, it is inadequate for some. It is likely that these patients are the ones who either have a substandard experience or receive excessive sedation, leading to increased adverse effects such as prolonged recovery or emesis.

Propofol traditionally is reserved for use by trained anesthesia professionals for several reasons. It easily results in deep sedation (especially when used as a sole agent). Additionally, state and institutional restrictions often limit who can administer propofol. Finally, the US Food and Drug Administration (FDA) package insert for propofol states that it "should be administered only by persons trained in the administration of general anesthesia and not involved in the conduct of the surgical/diagnostic procedure,"[7] imparting some potential medicolegal risk. Although the exact amount is debatable, it is certain that anesthesia-directed sedation (monitored anesthesia care or MAC) for routine endoscopic sedation involves some increased cost. Because propofol has many advantages to a benzodiazepine and opiate combination, alternative delivery models have been explored that use propofol for endoscopy without the involvement of anesthesia professionals, despite the potential impediments. These models include nurses trained in propofol sedation (nurse-administered propofol sedation or NAPS), low-dose propofol regimens that use propofol with other agents (usually opiates and benzodiazepine) to target moderate sedation (balanced propofol sedation or BPS), and robotic propofol administration (Sedasys, now off of the market). All of these practices that do not involve an anesthesia provider have come under the umbrella of endoscopist-directed sedation (EDS).[8] Effectiveness of EDS is similar or better in terms of patient satisfaction and recovery compared with moderate sedation.[9] There is no evidence to compare it directly to MAC, but effectiveness should be similar.

QUALITY, SAFETY, AND OUTCOMES

Sedation and anesthesia for lower endoscopy is generally safe.[9] However, many of the risks inherent to these procedures are sedation related.[10] EDS has been extensively evaluated as an alternate delivery model to propofol administered by anesthesia personnel. Multiple studies have examined deep sedation administered by nurses under the direction of the endoscopist or balanced propofol, in which small doses of opiates and benzodiazepines are used in conjunction with propofol to target moderate sedation. These studies have concluded that EDS for routine endoscopy is feasible and safe.[11] It is difficult to argue at this point that this practice is unsound.

Although EDS alone appears safe, a recent meta-analysis reviewed studies to evaluate the risk of cardiopulmonary events in patients receiving propofol versus other sedation for endoscopy and found no difference in rates of complications between different sedatives even when stratified by anesthesia versus nonanesthesia delivery.[12] In addition, several recent large database studies have evaluated the safety of sedation for endoscopy to determine if there is a safety difference between anesthetist-directed propofol sedation and endoscopist-directed moderate sedation. An evaluation of a large Medicare database assessed 165,527 lower endoscopic procedures in 100,539 patients and divided them into 2 groups: 35,128 procedures with anesthesia services (presumably received propofol) and 130,399 procedures without additional anesthesia services (presumably moderate sedation administered by the endoscopy team). The results revealed a small but statistically significant increase in aspiration in the anesthesia group but no change in the incidence of perforation or splenic injury. There was some effort to ensure that the groups did not differ in illness severity based on coding of comorbidities. It is possible that deeper sedation imparts a small increase in aspiration risk due to impairment of airway reflexes. However, uncontrolled confounders may have affected the results, as some patients receiving anesthesia services may be inherently at higher aspiration risk (eg, those with obesity or chronic opiate use).

A 2016 study sought to define the risk related to anesthesia services during colonoscopy.[13] The authors used a proprietary administrative database to identify over 3.1 million colonoscopies performed between 2008 and 2011 in patients between 40 to 64 years of age and divided the patients into 2 groups: 1 group receiving sedation care with anesthesia services (likely signifying sedation with propofol) and 1 group without (likely receiving moderate sedation with a benzodiazepine/opiate combination). In this database, 34.4% of patients had colonoscopy performed with anesthesia services. Overall complications, which included both potentially sedation-related (eg, pneumonia or aspiration) and not sedation-related (eg, postpolypectomy hemorrhage, perforation during polypectomy, or abdominal pain), were increased by 13% in those receiving anesthesia-directed care. There were no complications that were not increased in the anesthesia services group. Unrecognized confounders, including inability to identify patients having higher-risk procedures and inability to accurately identify patients with increased comorbidity (98.4% of patients in each group had no recognized significant comorbidities) may help explain the difference, as complex patients having complicated procedures and increased comorbidities may predispose to anesthesia-directed care.

A third database study published in 2017 evaluated 1.38 million procedures (a mixture of upper endoscopy and colonoscopy) in the Clinical Outcomes Research Initiative National Endoscopic Database. These procedures were stratified by the presence or not of an anesthesiologist and used a propensity score model to create a pseudorandomization. The overall rate of serious adverse events (SAEs) was similar for colonoscopy whether an anesthetist was involved or not (although SAEs were slightly but significantly higher for upper endoscopy when receiving anesthesia-directed care).[14] Although it may be debatable whether these 3 studies document a true risk to anesthesia-provided sedation, there was no evidence that care without anesthesia services was riskier.

Another potential advantage of sedation would be improved procedural outcomes. It has been postulated that sedation may improve quality of lower endoscopy since the patient is more comfortable, and the endoscopist may be able to complete a more thorough examination. A 2012 study evaluated the effect of sedation or no sedation on the quality of colonoscopy. The authors used an Austrian database that included data on 52,506 screening colonoscopies covering 196 endoscopy units. The practice in Austria is to offer the patient sedation if he or she wants it for colonoscopy. In this study, approximately 86% of patients received some type of sedation, but the exact type and agent used were not known. The use of sedation was not associated with an increase in adenoma detection rates. There was a slight increase in the cecal intubation rate with sedation, but sex and age explained most of the inability to reach the cecum. Other colonoscopy studies have not found significant differences in cecal intubation or polyp detection rate in sedated versus unsedated patients.[3,15–17]

Some experts have suggested that deep sedation may facilitate greater polyp detection rates due to better procedural conditions. A 2011 randomized study of 520 patients using midazolam and pethidine to target moderate versus deep sedation did not reveal a difference in detection rate.[18] This study did not have a propofol arm, and all sedation was controlled by the endoscopy team. Three retrospective studies[19–21] specifically evaluated propofol use and polyp detection rates with no apparent differences except in one study, which found an increase in large polyp detection with deep sedation but no difference overall. The data to date do not appear to show any outcome improvement for screening colonoscopy with deep sedation with or without propofol as compared to moderate sedation. The effect of sedation depth on more advanced procedures, such as endoscopic mucosal resection or endoscopic submucosal dissection, is not known at this time. However, these time-intensive advanced procedures may be more dependent on good operating conditions to obtain optimal outcomes.

UTILIZATION, COST, AND REIMBURSEMENT

Lower endoscopic procedures can be performed anywhere on the sedation spectrum, from no sedation to general anesthesia. Patients who previously have not tolerated moderate sedation or who use opiates chronically should receive deep sedation. Other groups of patients may benefit from anesthesia care, including those with significant comorbidities (ASA class 3 or higher), elevated body mass index (BMI), obstructive sleep apnea, known or suspected difficult airway, higher medical acuity such as active bleeding or hemodynamic instability, or those undergoing procedures of higher complexity and/or significant length. General anesthesia with active airway management should be reserved for specific rare situations based on patient comorbidities, acuity or procedural length, and complexity. Unfortunately, data on specific patient or procedural factors for lower endoscopy that would suggest an advantage of one sedation regimen over another are sparse. Two large retrospective database studies have found increased cardiopulmonary risk for colonoscopy in patients with ASA class 3 and above,[22,23] but whether this risk can be mitigated by the use of anesthesia services is unclear.

As previously mentioned, the use of anesthesia providers in endoscopic procedures has been steadily increasing. Although it would be logical and cost-effective to select the appropriate level of sedation care based on patient and procedural factors, the use of anesthesia services for discretionary lower endoscopic procedures is driven by several other factors. The favorable profile of propofol over other agents is likely the primary reason, but other causes include substantial regulatory and legal barriers to

EDS. From the endoscopist's perspective, there has been minimal reason to push for EDS until recently, as there was no financial incentive to encourage this practice. Additionally, there are some levels of hassle and legal risk. Recent reimbursement patterns have favored anesthesiologist involvement in routine colonoscopy. Thus far, many private insurers cover separate anesthesia care for lower endoscopy. In addition, CMS rules surrounding reimbursement for anesthesia services were clarified in 2015 to eliminate cost sharing for anesthesia for screening colonoscopy, which allows Medicare to be billed directly for these services in addition to the actual colonoscopy. New changes for 2017 may again change the financial incentives, as CMS has removed reimbursement for EDS (which was bundled into colonoscopy procedure codes) if an anesthesiologist is involved. This will lower the payment for colonoscopies that utilize anesthetist-directed sedation care. Although the present regulatory and legal environments continue to favor increasing demand for anesthetist-directed care for routine procedures, shifts in reimbursement may be less favorable to this practice.

The cost to the overall health care system of increasing use of anesthesia providers may be substantial. An evaluation in 2012 estimated that the providing anesthesia services for half of all colonoscopies would cost an additional 4.5 billion dollars over 10 years in the United States over EDS.[24] As previously discussed, there is no evidence that this increased cost leads to a reduction in significant sedation-related complications or improved clinical outcomes for lower endoscopy. It remains to be seen whether payers will continue to provide reimbursement for discretionary anesthesia care in the present financial environment.

SUMMARY

Deep sedation with propofol has clear advantages for lower endoscopic procedures, but these appear to be limited to improved satisfaction among patients and providers and increased efficiency in terms of readiness for discharge. There does not appear to be any advantage to depth of sedation in terms of procedural quality as defined by polyp detection or improvement in safety. When the sedation is directed by an anesthesiologist, overall costs increase, and this practice pattern is being increasingly utilized in the United States even for low-risk lower endoscopic procedures. The advantage of propofol may be achieved in specific low-risk patients having simple lower endoscopy by the use of endoscopist-directed sedation, but instituting this practice faces many institutional and regulatory hurdles. Some patients may tolerate colonoscopy with no sedation, which also can reduce complications and cost. For complex procedures or higher-risk patients, anesthesiologist involvement may be beneficial. In an ideal system, anesthesiologist-directed care would be reserved for higher-risk patients or complex procedures, with the option for EDS or no sedation for the remainder.

REFERENCES

1. ASA Continuum of Depth of Sedation. Approved by the ASA House of Delegates on October 27, 2004, and amended on October 21, 2009. Available at: asahq. org. Accessed February 1, 2017.
2. Rex DK, Imperiale TF, Portish V. Patients willing to try colonoscopy without sedation: associated clinical factors and results of a randomized controlled trial. Gastrointest Endosc 1999;49:554–9.
3. Petrini JL, Egan JV, Hahn WV. Unsedated colonoscopy: patient characteristics and satisfaction in a community-based endoscopy unit. Gastrointest Endosc 2009;69:567–72.

4. Predmore Z, Nie X, Main R, et al. Anesthesia service use during outpatient gastroenterology procedures continued to increase from 2010 to 2013 and potentially discretionary spending remained high. Am J Gastroenterol 2017;112:297–302.

5. Singh H, Poluha W, Cheang M, et al. Propofol for sedation in Colonoscopy. Cochrane Database Syst Rev 2008;4:1–65.

6. Patel S, Vargo JJ, Khandwala F, et al. Deep sedation occurs frequently during elective endoscopy with meperidine and midazolam. Am J Gastroenterol 2005; 100:2689–95.

7. Diprivan (propofol) injectable emulsion, USP. Available at: http://www.accessdata. fda.gov/drugsatfda_docs/label/2014/019627s062lbl.pdf. Accessed January 15, 2017.

8. Rex DK. Endoscopist-directed propofol. Gastrointest Endosc Clin N Am 2016;26: 485–92.

9. Vargo JJ, Cohen LB, Rex DK, et al. Position statement: nonanesthesiologist administration of propofol for GI endoscopy. Am J Gastroenterol 2009;104:2886–92.

10. Ko CW, Dominitz JA. Complications of colonoscopy: magnitude and management. Gastrointest Endosc Clin N Am 2010;20:659–71.

11. Rex DK, Deenadayalu VP, Eid E, et al. Endoscopist-directed administration of propofol: a worldwide experience. Gastroenterology 2009;137:1229–37.

12. Wadha V, Issa D, Garg S, et al. Similar risk of cardiopulmonary adverse events between propofol and traditional anesthesia for gastrointestinal endoscopy: a systematic review and meta-analysis. Clin Gastroenterol Hepat 2017;15:194–206.

13. Wernli KJ, Brenner AT, Rutter CM, et al. Risks associated with anesthesia services during colonoscopy. Gastroenterology 2016;150:888–94.

14. Vargo JJ, Niklewski PJ, Williams JL, et al. Patient safety during sedation by anesthesia professionals during routine upper endoscopy and colonoscopy: an analysis of 1.38 million procedures. Clin Endosc 2017;85:101–8.

15. Eckardt VF, Kanzler G, Willems D, et al. Colonoscopy without premedication versus barium enema: a comparison of patient discomfort. Gastrointest Endosc 1996;44:177–80.

16. Takahashi Y, Tanaka H, Kinjo M, et al. Sedation-free colonoscopy. Dis Colon Rectum 2005;48:855–9.

17. Leung JW, Mann S, Leung FW. Options for screening colonoscopy without sedation: a pilot study in United States veterans. Aliment Pharmacol Ther 2007;26: 627–31.

18. Paspatis GA, Tribonias G, Manolaraki MM, et al. Deep sedation compared with moderate sedation in polyp detection during colonoscopy: a randomized controlled trial. Colorectal Dis 2011;13:e137–44.

19. Metwally M, Agresty N, Hale WB, et al. Conscious or unconscious: The impact of sedation choice on colon adenoma detection. World J Gastroenterol 2011;17:3912–5.

20. Wang A, Hoda KM, Holub JL, et al. Does level of sedation impact detection of advanced neoplasia. Dig Dis Sci 2010;55:2337–43.

21. Nakshabendi R, Berry AC, Munoz JM. Choice of sedation and its impact on adenoma detection rate in screening colonoscopies. Ann Gastroenterol 2016;29:50–5.

22. Sharma VK, Nguyen CC, Crowell MD, et al. A national study of cardiopulmonary unplanned events after GI endoscopy. Gastrointest Endosc 2007;66:27–34.

23. Warren JL, Klabunde CN, Mariotto AB, et al. Adverse events after outpatient colonoscopy in the Medicare population. Ann Intern Med 2009;150:849–57.

24. Hassan C, Rex DK, Cooper GS, et al. Endoscopist-directed propofol administration versus anesthesiologist assistance for colorectal cancer screening: a cost-effectiveness analysis. Endoscopy 2012;44:456–64.

Interventional Pulmonology

David M. DiBardino, MD[a],*, Andrew R. Haas, MD, PhD[a], Richard C. Month, MD[b]

KEYWORDS

- Bronchoscopy • Jet ventilation • Total intravenous anesthesia
- Interventional pulmonology

KEY POINTS

- Advances in interventional pulmonology techniques allow for the care of patients of significantly higher acuity. These patients can be best cared for in a well-planned multidisciplinary fashion.
- Airway access in interventional pulmonology patients is often a shared responsibility between the pulmonologist and anesthesiologist. Commonly, airways are managed with advanced airway devices such as laryngeal masks or endotracheal tubes.
- Anesthetic techniques vary widely depending on the length and nature of the procedure and the acuity of the patient. Most commonly, these patients are anesthetized with a total intravenous anesthetic technique.
- Management of these patients is commonly complicated by issues such as central airway obstruction, tracheal stenosis, and the need for jet ventilation or rigid bronchoscopy.

Bronchoscopy presents a unique challenge and need for collaboration between anesthesia providers and bronchoscopists. The approach to topical anesthesia, analgesia, and sedation needs to be customized based on the complexity, duration, and setting of the procedure.[1] Although many straightforward bronchoscopies can be performed with topical anesthesia and moderate sedation, recent advances in diagnostic and therapeutic bronchoscopy have increased procedural complexity and length. Consequently, increasing numbers of institutions prefer to perform interventional pulmonary procedures using the combination of topical anesthesia and total intravenous anesthesia (TIVA) in the operating room. This approach may maximize both patient satisfaction and procedural conditions.[2,3] In addition, cultivation of a team of anesthesia

Disclosure Statement: The authors have nothing to disclose.
[a] Section of Interventional Pulmonology, Division of Pulmonary, Allergy and Critical Care, University of Pennsylvania, 3400 Spruce Street, 839 West Gates Building, Philadelphia, PA 19104, USA; [b] Department of Anesthesiology and Critical Care, University of Pennsylvania, 3400 Spruce Street, 7th Floor Ravdin Building, Philadelphia, PA 19104, USA
* Corresponding author.
E-mail address: David.DiBardino@uphs.upenn.edu

Anesthesiology Clin 35 (2017) 687–699
http://dx.doi.org/10.1016/j.anclin.2017.08.004
1932-2275/17/© 2017 Elsevier Inc. All rights reserved.

anesthesiology.theclinics.com

providers with expertise and interest in complex bronchoscopy and airway procedures can foster team work and collaboration, as well as maximize quality and procedural outcomes.

The bronchoscopy team must work together in each phase of the procedure to ensure patient safety and to allow completion of a quality bronchoscopy. Airway access may change depending on the type of procedure planned and must be discussed before each case. Intraprocedural difficulties with ventilation, airway pressure, and sedation may arise that need to be addressed as a team. Additionally, although outside the scope of this review, patients with lung disease are often compromised after bronchoscopy and need multidisciplinary recovery care. The goal of this review is to highlight an approach to these common challenges faced by anesthesiologists and interventional pulmonologists during advanced bronchoscopy.

AIRWAY ACCESS

Before each procedure, an airway plan should be discussed between the anesthesia providers and interventional pulmonary team. A morning huddle to review all cases planned for the day can allow both the bronchoscopy and anesthesia teams to anticipate and to prepare for potentially complex cases requiring special airway management considerations.

Supraglottic Airway Devices

Many advanced bronchoscopy programs have defaulted to supraglottic airway devices, typically a laryngeal mask, as the standard approach to allow full airway access and to provide ventilator support. By convention, a size 4, 4.5, or 5 laryngeal mask is used in men and a size 3, 3.5, or 4 in women provided there was a normal physical examination. This approach has been reported as a safe option in many contexts in the interventional pulmonary literature that includes complex airway interventions.[2–7] This is especially relevant with endobronchial ultrasound-guided transbronchial needle aspiration in which the laryngeal mask allows full bronchoscope access to image and to sample the paratracheal lymph nodes.

Proper laryngeal mask placement can be confirmed by direct bronchoscopic visualization, and adjustments to its position or interventions to treat other causes of hypoventilation (eg, laryngospasm) can be undertaken before the procedure fully commences.

Endotracheal Tube

Traditional endotracheal tube (ETT) placement is always an option to facilitate bronchoscopy for patients with predictably difficult mask ventilation, who fail laryngeal mask, or who have a history of inability to ventilate with a laryngeal mask. ETT intubation should be considered in a patient who presents for bronchoscopy with traditional contraindications to a supraglottic airway, such as oropharyngeal or proximal esophageal disease, large hiatal hernia, esophageal motility disorder, significant or untreated gastroesophageal reflux disease, or complex supraglottic airway anatomy from malignancy, prior surgery, and/or radiation. In addition, relative complications to laryngeal mask may also lead to endotracheal intubation. These include anticipation of a prolonged procedure, significant obesity, or comorbid conditions in which hypoventilation would have significant risk (eg, severe pulmonary arterial hypertension). However, because laryngeal mask utilization has been slowly liberalizing and safety is being demonstrated in more varied patient populations, the final decision regarding airway should rest in the hands of the care team, taking into account specific patient and procedural factors.[8]

If endotracheal intubation is chosen, using a tube with an adequate inner diameter is crucial to accommodate the diagnostic bronchoscopes to be used and to allow appropriate ventilation (see later discussion).

Rigid Bronchoscopy

Many interventional pulmonary practices incorporate rigid bronchoscopy in select patients. The rigid bronchoscope simultaneously allows a stable airway, the largest available working channel for multiple instruments, and a ventilating lumen. These advantages can enhance safety, efficacy, and efficiency of procedures in which central airway obstruction with tumor or a foreign body is anticipated. Other procedures, such as silicone stent placement, also require the use of the rigid bronchoscope.[9] Despite its many advantages, the rigid bronchoscope does not allow for a closed ventilator circuit. Patients can be managed with either jet ventilation or traditional ventilator modes with mouth packing (see later discussion).

When a rigid bronchoscopy is anticipated, discussions between the anesthesia team and bronchoscopist center on the safety of paralysis, anticipated use of jet ventilation, and predicted pulmonary reserve. Before rigid bronchoscope intubation, a flexible bronchoscope airway inspection via a laryngeal mask allows the bronchoscopist to plan and to communicate with the anesthesia team regarding the potential components and complexity of the rigid bronchoscopy that might require special considerations. After confirming the necessity of rigid bronchoscopy, the patient is prepared with a paralytic (unless contraindicated), proper intubation position, preoxygenation, and denitrogenation using the laryngeal mask. During this time, the presence of all necessary equipment for the rigid intubation, jet ventilation, volume ventilation, mouth packing, teeth protection, mouth suction, conventional endotracheal ventilation, and mask ventilation supplies are confirmed. The laryngeal mask is removed and rigid intubation commences once all members of the bronchoscopy and anesthesia teams are ready. On successful rigid bronchoscope airway intubation, the rigid bronchoscope is connected to a jet ventilator using a specially designed luer lock adapter (**Fig. 1**), whereas traditional ventilator modes are used only if the patient cannot tolerate jet ventilation.

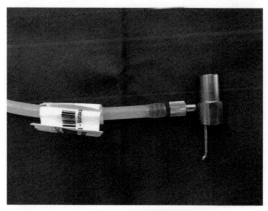

Fig. 1. Luer lock device connected to jet ventilator tubing. The metal prong feeds the jet stream directly down the rigid bronchoscope barrel.

Tracheostomy Patients

Patients with tracheostomy tubes often require bronchoscopy. There are several options for airway access, depending on how recently the tracheostomy was placed and on the size of the tracheal lumen. A stable and mature tracheostomy tube can be removed and replaced with a larger inner diameter ETT that will accommodate the bronchoscope to be used for the procedure. The tracheostomy tube is then replaced after conclusion of the procedure. A standard ETT can be shortened above the pilot balloon to allow maximal maneuverability while maintaining ETT and bronchoscope control. If endobronchial ultrasound is needed, a 9.0-mm internal diameter standard ETT is preferred to allow adequate ventilation around the larger endobronchial ultrasound bronchoscope (**Fig. 2**). Generally, the outer diameters of standard tracheostomy tubes create stomas large enough accommodate the outer diameters of 8.0-mm and 9.0-mm inner diameter ETTs with gentle pressure during insertion. As an example, a Shiley 6.0-mm inner tube has a 10.1-mm outer diameter that is large enough to accommodate the 12.1-mm outer diameter of a 9.0-mm inner diameter Mallinckrodt ETT.

In some situations, patients may present for bronchoscopy with recent tracheostomy tube placement in which a mature stoma has not formed, thus making tube removal and manipulation unsafe. Despite a lack of evidence, consensus guidelines suggest a surgical tracheostomy tube should not be replaced before 3 days and a percutaneous dilational tracheostomy should not be replaced before 10 days.[10] In these circumstances, consideration should be given to delaying the procedure if clinically possible. If the bronchoscopy is necessary, it is important to choose a

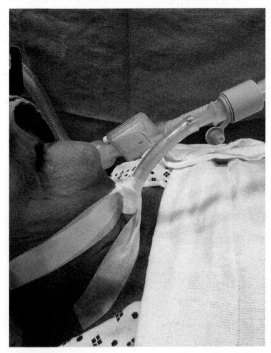

Fig. 2. ETT being used within a tracheostomy stoma. Shown is a 9.0-mm tube cut short to enhance control of the bronchoscope.

bronchoscope that will allow simultaneous ventilation and completion of the bronchoscopy goals. If the patient is not ventilator-dependent, the inner cannula can be removed to allow for a larger airway lumen to pass the bronchoscope.

Tracheoesophageal Fistula

Special consideration is needed for tracheoesophageal fistula (TEF) patients who require an airway or who undergo a bronchoscopy or endoscopy with anesthesia and positive pressure ventilation. Intraprocedural ventilation must be achieved using an airway above the defect to allow adequate access to the trachea for full inspection and potential intervention. In addition, bronchoscopic-guided tube placement is essential to avoid malposition of the airway into the fistula or to prevent further TEF extension from ETT insertion. Ventilatory capacity can be lost through the TEF if it is large enough. These cases require close communication and management with the anesthesia team. In patients who are not endotracheally intubated due to respiratory failure, a laryngeal mask provides full access to the trachea, allowing assessment of the TEF location and severity.

Central Airway Obstruction

Interventional pulmonary procedures done in the operating room may involve some degree of central airway obstruction. These cases may be uniquely challenging, depending on the degree of airway obstruction, the degree of respiratory compromise, and the degree of the underlying pulmonary reserve of the patient. Moreover, the therapeutic interventions may precipitate bleeding that can affect visualization and/or ventilation. If expertise exists, rigid bronchoscopy utilization allows for the largest and most effective tools and simultaneous airway control and ventilation.[9] For central airway obstructions involving only the right or left mainstem bronchus, another benefit of rigid bronchoscopy is isolating the airway with the pathologic condition. Ventilating side ports allow for ventilation from the jet stream to pass into the unaffected mainstem bronchus with minimal soilage of the nonintubated mainstem airway (**Fig. 3**).

Central airway obstruction may cause respiratory failure, requiring endotracheal intubation before the therapeutic bronchoscopy can be performed. These patients need careful conversion to rigid bronchoscopy, followed by the re-establishment of a secure airway for ventilator weaning. This can be challenging because the prior insertion and presence of an ETT can precipitate arytenoid and glottis edema that

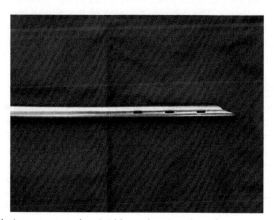

Fig. 3. Side ventilation ports on the rigid bronchoscope barrel.

can make further airway access difficult. In this circumstance, an option is to insert the rigid bronchoscope along the ETT to visualize the glottis structures, and then remove the ETT slowly as the rigid bronchoscope is advanced. Alternatively, an airway exchange catheter that allows jet ventilation can be exchanged for the ETT to allow airway access while the rigid bronchoscope intubation is performed. If rigid bronchoscope intubation is problematic, the exchange catheter may be used to jet ventilate the patient and to reinsert a new ETT without losing airway access. In central airway obstruction caused by a friable, bleeding tumor, blind insertion of an airway exchange catheter into the airway should be avoided to prevent further trauma and bleeding. Furthermore, if a tracheal obstruction requires tracheal stent placement and the patient requires further ventilator support, re-establishing a secure airway before transfer to the intensive care unit requires bronchoscopic guidance. After rigid extubation, these patients can be conventionally reintubated; however, the proper placement of the ETT must be directly visualized to ensure the ETT does not dislodge the airway stent. This consideration is particularly important for upper tracheal stents, and requires careful coordination with the anesthesia team.

APPROACHES TO SEDATION

Several approaches to sedation or anesthesia exist for airway examination. These range from awake methods, through moderate and deep sedation, to general anesthesia. Each approach has risks and benefits that must be considered in regard to the specific procedure and patient, as well as in terms of the availability of resources and staff.

Awake Methods

Awake methods, those without accompanying intravenous sedation, may be used for a narrow population of patients and procedures; however, due to the highly reactive nature of the posterior pharynx and vocal cords, these procedures are typically not tolerated for an extended period of time. Such procedures are always accompanied with applied topical local anesthesia (see later discussion).

Procedures that lend themselves to awake methods include evaluation of the supraglottis or vocal cords, evaluation of the trachea, or rapid airway evaluation. In addition, a narrow group of emergency procedures may be performed under an awake topicalized method to avoid the respiratory depression that accompanies intravenous sedation or general anesthesia. The primary benefits of the awake method are that the patient is able respond to command and the airways can be evaluated in a dynamic, rather than a static, state. Procedures of any extended length of time will typically require some additional sedation for patient comfort and to facilitate the examination.

Moderate (Conscious) Sedation

Moderate sedation is defined by the American Society of Anesthesiologists as "a drug-induced depression of consciousness during which patients respond purposefully to verbal commands, either alone or accompanied by light tactile stimulation."[11] Moderate sedation is a common modality used for short and minimally invasive procedures. It has wide utility in the bronchoscopy suite for several procedures that do not lead to significant pain or reflex activation, and do not require significant akinesis. These procedures include basic airway evaluation and pleural drain placement. Moderate sedation is typically performed using a combination of short-acting anxiolytics (most commonly midazolam) and opioids (most commonly fentanyl). However, several other medications, including low-dose propofol or dexmedetomidine, may be used to reach this level of anesthesia.

Although, by definition, moderate sedation is well-tolerated and maintains airway patency, the provider must always be prepared for rescue from deep sedation or general anesthesia and be prepared to treat hypoventilation.

Deep Sedation

Deep sedation implies a more advanced anesthetic state than that of moderate sedation; in it, the patient loses the ability to be easily aroused and requires repeated or painful stimulation to respond purposefully.[11] Deep sedation may lead to the inability to maintain airway patency or adequate ventilation; therefore, the ability to identify and rescue from general anesthesia is a must during deep sedation. For these reasons, the *Hospital Anesthesia Services Condition of Participation* limits administration of deep sedation to a medical doctor, doctor of osteopathy, nurse anesthetist, anesthesiologist assistant, or other physician qualified to administer anesthesia under state law.

Deep sedation may be used for longer or more invasive procedures in which maintenance of respiration is desirable but akinesis is not required. Most commonly, deep sedation is achieved with a sedative or hypnotic by infusion (most commonly propofol 50–80 μg/kg/min).

General Anesthesia

With growing frequency, interventional pulmonology procedures are performed under general anesthesia. General anesthesia allows for a more secure airway management because a laryngeal mask or ETT may be inserted. It also allows akinesis, allowing for finer control of placement of the scope for imaging or biopsy.

Because suction through the bronchoscope and interruptions of the breathing circuit typically preclude the use of volatile anesthetics, the most common modality for achieving general anesthesia in the bronchoscopy suite is through TIVA. Techniques typically involve a sedative or hypnotic infusion (most commonly propofol 100–150 μg/kg/min) and an ultrashort-acting opioid to assist with akinesis (most commonly remifentanil 0.1–0.2 μg/kg/min). Hypotension is common with TIVA administration; therefore, it is not uncommon to add a vasopressor, such as phenylephrine 50 to 100 μg/min, to the anesthetic.

In circumstances in which akinesis is absolutely required (eg, rigid bronchoscopy, in which movement could be life-threatening), the addition of a nondepolarizing muscle relaxant (vecuronium, rocuronium) may be considered. Residual neuromuscular blockade can lead to hypoventilation and postprocedure respiratory collapse; therefore, reversal of neuromuscular blockade to a train-of-four ratio greater than 90% should assured before emergence. The selective neuromuscular relaxant binding agent sugammadex (2–4 mg/kg) is gaining growing acceptance as a safe, rapid, and effective way to ensure this reversal.[12]

Topical Anesthesia

Topical anesthetic use is vital to anesthetic and procedural success regardless of the intravenous sedation plan.[13] Various topical anesthetics may be used in a variety of concentrations. A balance between copious fluid in the airway and high doses of anesthetic is achieved with 2% lidocaine. Higher concentrations, such as 4% lidocaine, may be used in nebulized form when anesthetizing the oropharynx. With TIVA it is not necessary to anesthetize the oropharynx with a topical agent.

At the vocal cords, topical lidocaine 2% should be administered via the bronchoscope to the glottis structures to quell the glottis and cough reflexes. It is important to maintain lidocaine dosage below the safety 5.0 to 7.0 mg/kg limit.[13]

Precautions in Critical Airway Obstruction

Critical tracheal stenosis

Patients with critical tracheal stenosis are among the most difficult to treat. Well-conditioned patients may present late in their disease state with a tracheal lumen of only several millimeters. Many of these stenoses are in the subglottic space or proximal trachea, precluding the ability to pass an ETT as a primary or salvage airway. Many times, minimal patency is only maintained by extrinsic muscle tone, and this may be lost during anesthetic induction regardless of whether a paralyzing agent is administered. During the preprocedural evaluation, the patient should be asked if they can lay flat. If the patient is unable to comply due to dyspnea, the airway is truly critical and management should only be handled by an expert multidisciplinary airway and anesthesia team. In patients with critical stenosis, there is no guarantee that positive pressure ventilation above the stenosis will be effective once the patient is under anesthesia. With judicious use of topical anesthesia and minimal sedation, a balloon dilation with or without mucosal incisions can be achieved with the patient upright, awake, and spontaneously breathing. This initial awake dilation achieves a safer tracheal luminal diameter to proceed with more conventional anesthesia and therapeutic intervention.

Mediastinal mass

Similar to the patient with a critical tracheal stenosis, a patient with a large anterior mediastinal mass may be inappropriate for general anesthesia because of their vulnerable airway. In these patients, there is particular concern that obliteration of airway and loss of thoracic muscle tone (with the use of paralytic agents) may result in rapid and life-threatening loss of the airway. The diagnostic and therapeutic approach to airway management must be contemplated carefully. Patient treatment may allow for a non-anesthesia biopsy approach (eg, image-guided percutaneous biopsy) or a biopsy location that does not require anesthesia. Should bronchoscopy remain the best biopsy approach, consider performing the procedure with topical anesthesia and minimal sedation with the patient breathing spontaneously. These patients also require careful consideration to vascular access and hemodynamics. The mediastinal mass may extrinsically compress the superior and/or inferior vena cava, making patients vulnerable to loss of preload after the administration of vasodilating anesthetic agents. This loss of preload may further lead to hemodynamic compromise and even cardiac arrest. Should this occur, this same vascular obstruction can make rapid advanced cardiac life support medication administration less effective.

Laryngospasm

Laryngospasm, a strong reflex closure of the vocal cords, is a complication of scope placement. Laryngospasm may lead to airway obstruction, hypoxia, and negative-pressure pulmonary edema. It is often a consequence of airway manipulation (either by scope or by airway device) before achieving adequate anesthetic depth. Avoiding this vigorous stimulus is an advantage of airway access using an ETT.

Laryngospasm will often present in a clinically overt way.[14] During bronchoscopy, the providers have an added advantage of examining the vocal cords when laryngospasm is suspected. Once confirmed, laryngospasm requires prompt action to deepen the level of anesthesia and increase the ventilator circuit driving pressure.

The patient's underlying pulmonary reserve dictates how urgent and aggressively to treat the laryngospasm. In patients who are able to maintain normal oxygen saturation, several basic steps can be used: additional topical anesthesia to the vocal cords, high-pressure assisted ventilation, and bolus intravenous sedation. If these measures fail or oxygen desaturation begins, low-dose succinylcholine (0.1 mg/kg) can be given. If these measures fail before the patient is able to be reoxygenated, the cords can be mechanically separated by gently pushing the bronchoscope past the posterior commissure of the vocal cords.

VENTILATION

Bronchoscopy is well-known to cause transient hypoxemia that can usually be overcome with supplemental oxygen administration.[15,16] The management of hypoxemic respiratory failure with supplemental oxygen is facilitated by the ventilator circuit with an artificial airway. However, acute hypercapnia due to hypoventilation likely occurs in all patients undergoing bronchoscopy to some degree.[17] Having a systematic approach to diagnosing and treating hypercapnia and hypoventilation is crucial when performing a procedure using moderate sedation, TIVA, or a laryngeal mask. Oxygen saturation alone is an inaccurate way to gauge ventilation when supplemental oxygen is being provided.[18] Measuring adequate ventilation with exhaled capnography or transcutaneous carbon dioxide (CO_2) measurement is a necessary monitor to supplement continuous pulse oximetry.

When hypoventilation is suspected based on objective measurement or subjective assessment of the patient, continuous, direct communication must take place between the anesthesia provider and the bronchoscopist. The bronchoscopist is able provide feedback on airway obstruction, including a vocal cord examination to rule out laryngospasm. The anesthesia provider is able to evaluate air leaks in the ventilator circuit. When using a laryngeal mask, poor mask fit is the most common reason for an air leak. Air leak may also be exacerbated by several factors that make any patient difficult to mask ventilate: supine position with abdominal obesity, decreased chest wall compliance, pre-existing lung disease being exacerbated by diagnostic techniques (eg, adding lavage fluid, bleeding), and increased airway resistance from luminal obstruction caused by either the bronchoscope or intrinsic airway disease. Most laryngeal mask-related hypoventilation may be overcome by the anesthesia team optimizing laryngeal mask position, cuff pressure, and by hand ventilation using high pressure. The procedure team is then able to confirm laryngeal mask position bronchoscopically. Should these approaches be ineffective to achieve adequate ventilation, the bronchoscopy team can increase the oropharyngeal resistance by closing the nostrils and mouth around the mask, as well as lifting the submental space into the cuff (**Fig. 4**). After position and fit have been optimized and reversible airway obstruction has been treated, continued hypoventilation despite hand ventilation is an indication to remove the bronchoscope from the airway. In the rare circumstance that these measures have all failed, the laryngeal mask should be removed, the patient mask ventilated, and endotracheal intubation undertaken. The threshold at which the supraglottic approach is abandoned is a matter of patient stability. Patients with hypoxemia or hemodynamic aberrancies are very likely to have significant hypercapnia and often unable to tolerate further mask troubleshooting.

Ventilation Using the Jet Ventilator

Hypoventilation is even more difficult to diagnose and treat during high-frequency jet ventilation. Exhaled CO_2 cannot be measured reliably without using a specialty device

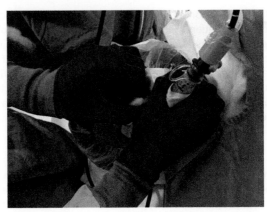

Fig. 4. Optimizing laryngeal mask airway seal by pinching the nares closed and elevating the submental space.

to sample tracheal gas or with transcutaneous measurement.[19–22] Serial arterial blood gas monitoring is an ideal, although often impractical, way to manage a patient on jet ventilation. However, using standard jet ventilator settings, continuous pulse oximetry, observing for chest rise, and minimizing the amount of time a patient requires jet ventilation usually achieves adequate ventilation in most patients.[9,21,23]

Significant hypoventilation using jet ventilation via the rigid bronchoscope with a frequency of 120 jets per minute, 100% oxygen, and a driving pressure between 25 and 30 psi occurs rarely outside of hypoxemia.[24] Therefore, pulse oximetry is used to indicate oxygenation and as a supplemental gauge of significant hypoventilation. When significant hypoventilation is suspected, several basic steps can be taken to improve hypercapnia and associated oxygen desaturation. The driving pressure of the jet ventilator may be increased within recommended limits.[23] The inspired oxygen may also be increased by replacing entrained room air with 100% oxygen. The rigid bronchoscope jet ventilator adapter is able accommodate standard ventilator extension tubing to provide extra oxygen (**Fig. 5**). This adjustment can only be expected to have modest benefit because inspired oxygen using jet ventilation approaches 80% to 90%.[23] Reverse Trendelenburg positioning can be used to improve chest wall compliance. Finally, the position of the rigid scope can be altered. Despite the ventilation ports allowing jet streams to escape outside of the rigid barrel, most of the oxygen is propelled forward through the barrel based on the relatively laminar flow of the jet stream.

If these measures have not improved oxygenation and increased ventilation, consider changing the mode of ventilation from jet ventilation to volume-controlled ventilation via the traditional ventilator circuit. This approach requires the previously mentioned connection using ventilator extension tubing and the standard rigid bronchoscope ventilator adapter (see **Fig. 5**). To ventilate effectively, all sources of air leak must be manually closed, including the oropharynx, nostrils, rigid barrel at the glottis, and the suction port of the rigid scope. The air leak from the nasopharynx and oropharynx requires pinching the nose and closing the mouth around the rigid bronchoscope, or by packing the oropharynx at the glottis to prevent air leaks. At this point, end-tidal CO_2 measurements should be monitored as mechanical or hand ventilation is initiated.

Vigilance is required when using the rigid bronchoscope with jet ventilation in patients with tracheal stenosis. Much of the open circuit may be closed when the rigid

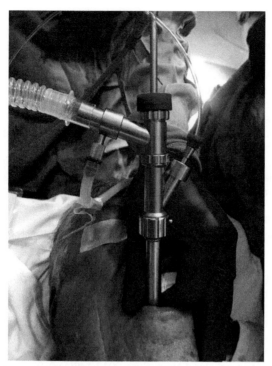

Fig. 5. Rigid barrel connected to the anesthesia circuit with extension tubing, as well as the jet ventilator via the luer lock adapter.

bronchoscope is passed beyond the stenosis. Preventing the air egress may lead to barotrauma. To prevent serious barotrauma, it is critical to ensure the ventilation circuit is open in some fashion, or to lower the jet ventilator pressure limit (the so-called pause pressure). Some investigators have advocated for a pause pressure near 5 to 10 millibar (~5–10 cm water) to avoid barotrauma in any circumstance.[23]

SUMMARY

Advances in diagnostic and therapeutic bronchoscopy have increased the length, duration, and complexity of bronchoscopy procedures. Many bronchoscopy programs have shifted from moderate sedation to deeper sedation and general anesthesia. Patient management in the bronchoscopy suite requires close collaboration between the anesthesia and primary bronchoscopy teams. Anesthesia support during the challenges of unique intraprocedural complications is key to quickly and effectively restoring the safety of the procedure. In this manner, successful diagnostic and/or therapeutic bronchoscopies can be performed to maximize the patient experience, comfort, safety, and outcome.

REFERENCES

1. Wahidi MM, Jain P, Jantz M, et al. American college of chest physicians consensus statement on the use of topical anesthesia, analgesia, and sedation during flexible bronchoscopy in adult patients. Chest 2011;140(5):1342–50.

2. Raafat H, Mahmoud A, Salem S. Comparison between bronchoscopy under general anesthesia using laryngeal mask airway and local anesthesia with conscious sedation: a patient-centered and operator-centered outcome. Egypt J Broncho 2014;8(2):128–37.

3. Yarmus LB, Akulian JA, Gilbert C, et al. Comparison of moderate versus deep sedation for endobronchial ultrasound transbronchial needle aspiration. Ann Am Thorac Soc 2013;10(2):121–6.

4. Qassem Z, Zeid F, Gress T. The safety of using laryngeal mask airways (LMA) in diagnostic fiber optic bronchoscopy. Chest 2009;139(4_MeetingAbstracts): 82S-a.

5. Bouaggad A, Bennani F, Al Harrar R, et al. Anesthesia for a patient with tracheal tumor using laryngeal mask airway. Anesth Analg 2006;103(1):258–9.

6. Chhetri DK, Long JL. Airway management and CO2 laser treatment of subglottic and tracheal stenosis using flexible bronchoscope and laryngeal mask anesthesia. Oper Tech Otolaryngol 2011;22(2):131–4.

7. Snow NJ, Massad MG, Geha AS, et al. Use of the laryngeal mask airway for diagnostic and interventional bronchoscopy. Chest 2004;126(4_MeetingAbstracts): 736S.

8. Verghese C, Brimacombe JR. Survey of laryngeal mask airway usage in 11,910 patients: safety and efficacy for conventional and nonconventional usage. Anesth Analg 1996;82:129–33.

9. Gorden JA. Rigid bronchoscopy. In: Ernst A, Herth FJF, editors. Principles and practice of interventional pulmonology. New York: Springer; 2013. p. 285–95.

10. Mitchell RB, Hussey HM, Setzen G, et al. Clinical consensus statement: tracheostomy care. Otolaryngol Head Neck Surg 2013;148(1):6–20.

11. American Society of Anesthesiologists. Practice guidelines for sedation and analgesia by non-anesthesiologists. Anesthesiology 2002;96:1004–17.

12. Pawlowski J. Anesthetic considerations for interventional pulmonology procedures. Curr Opin Anesthesiol 2013;26:6–12.

13. Pawlowski J. Moderate and deep sedation techniques. In: Ernst A, Herth FJF, editors. Principles and practice of interventional pulmonology. New York: Springer; 2013. p. 63–72.

14. Visvanathan T, Kluger MT, Webb RK, et al. Crisis management during anaesthesia: laryngospasm. Qual Saf Health Care 2005;14(3):e3.

15. Schnabel RM, van der Velden K, Osinski A, et al. Clinical course and complications following diagnostic bronchoalveolar lavage in critically ill mechanically ventilated patients. BMC Pulm Med 2015;15:107.

16. Chhajed PN, Glanville AR. Management of hypoxemia during flexible bronchoscopy. Clin Chest Med 2003;24(3):511–6.

17. Chhajed PN, Rajasekaran R, Kaegi B, et al. Measurement of combined oximetry and cutaneous capnography during flexible bronchoscopy. ERJ 2006;28(2): 386–90.

18. Fu ES, Downs JB, Schweiger JW, et al. Supplemental oxygen impairs detection of hypoventilation by pulse oximetry. Chest 2004;126(5):1552–8.

19. Desruennes E, Bourgain JL, Mamelle G, et al. Airway obstruction and high-frequency jet ventilation during laryngoscopy. Ann Otol Rhinol Laryngol 1991; 100(11):922–7.

20. Bourgain JL, McGee K, Cosset MF, et al. Carbon dioxide monitoring during high frequency jet ventilation for direct laryngoscopy. Br J Anaesth 1990;64(3):327–30.

21. Biro P, Layer M, Wiedemann K, et al. Carbon dioxide elimination during high-frequency jet ventilation for rigid bronchoscopy. Br J Anaesth 2000;84(5):635–7.

22. Hautmann H, Gamarra F, Henke M, et al. High frequency jet ventilation in interventional fiberoptic bronchoscopy. Anesth Analg 2000;90(6):1436–40.
23. Putz L, Mayné A, Dincq AS. Jet ventilation during rigid bronchoscopy in adults: a focused review. Biomed Res Int 2016;2016:4234861.
24. Cheng Q, Zhang J, Wang H, et al. Effect of acute hypercapnia on outcomes and predictive risk factors for complications among patients receiving bronchoscopic interventions under general anesthesia. PLoS One 2015;10(7):e0130771.

Pediatric Anesthesia Considerations for Interventional Radiology

Olivia Nelson, MD[a], Philip D. Bailey Jr, DO, MBA[b],*

KEYWORDS

- Pediatric anesthesia • Interventional radiology (IR)
- Non–operating room anesthesia (NORA) • Vascular access • Sclerotherapy
- Chemosurgery • Radiation safety

KEY POINTS

- Non–operating room diagnostics and procedures comprise an increasing volume of pediatric anesthesia practice; considerations for pediatric patients are different than adults owing to age and maturity.
- Pediatric patients often require general anesthesia for interventional radiology (IR); planning should consider specific requirements of the procedure.
- Pediatric patients with oncologic processes may present for biopsies and vascular access; some may have anterior mediastinal masses making preprocedural risk assessment and planning vital.
- Sclerotherapy for vascular malformations is a lengthy procedure requiring patient immobility and injection of sclerosing agents with potential adverse effects.
- Risk factors include effects of medications and radiographic contrast media, procedure-specific risks, and exposure of patients and personnel to ionizing radiation.

INTRODUCTION

Anesthesiologists are increasingly called on to care for pediatric patients undergoing diagnostic imaging and procedures in locations outside of the traditional operating room theater in what has come to be known as non–operating room anesthesia locations. Indeed, in most large pediatric hospitals approximately 30% to 40% of the case volume is accounted for in these non–operating room anesthesia venues. These cases

Disclosure Statement: The author's have no conflicts of interest to declare. Support for this article was provided solely from institutional and/or departmental resources.
[a] Department of Anesthesiology and Critical Care Medicine, The Children's Hospital of Philadelphia, 9th Floor, 3401 Civic Center Boulevard, Philadelphia, PA 19104, USA; [b] Department of Anesthesiology and Critical Care Medicine, Perelman School of Medicine, The University of Pennsylvania, The Children's Hospital of Philadelphia, 9th Floor, 3401 Civic Center Boulevard, Philadelphia, PA 19104, USA
* Corresponding author.
E-mail address: Baileyp@email.chop.edu

Anesthesiology Clin 35 (2017) 701–714
http://dx.doi.org/10.1016/j.anclin.2017.08.003
1932-2275/17/© 2017 Elsevier Inc. All rights reserved.

anesthesiology.theclinics.com

can range from short diagnostic imaging studies to significantly longer and more invasive intravascular procedures in interventional radiology (IR). There is significant institutional variation in how these cases are approached, with relatively few studies on optimal management.

There are concerns specific to pediatric patients that the anesthesia provider should take into account when preparing the anesthetic plan. Such planning should take into account the patient's age and comorbidities. Other important considerations include the type of procedure and the constraints of the non–operating room environment that may limit access to the patient or familiar equipment and personnel. Specific procedural considerations include the need for breath holding, patient immobility, and the duration of the procedure, as well as the possibility of certain procedure-specific complications. Patient immobility can be important for safety, particularly for endovascular procedures, and for minimizing doses of radiation for diagnostic studies. In this review, we address specific considerations in planning for IR procedures that are frequently performed in the pediatric population.

PEDIATRIC AND PATIENT-SPECIFIC CONSIDERATIONS

Providers administering anesthesia to pediatric patients must consider each child's ability to cooperate reliably during the procedure as well as their patient's age and any cognitive impairments. Owing to these constraints, children often require general anesthesia for procedures that could be performed under moderate sedation for adult patients. Additionally, medical comorbidities may limit the patient's ability to undergo procedures with sedation safely and comfortably, making general anesthesia the best option.

Oncology Patients

Pediatric oncology patients can present for a variety of IR procedures during the course of their initial diagnosis and treatment. These can include biopsy to allow tissue diagnosis and treatment planning, and lumbar puncture to assess for possible spread of malignancy and administration of intrathecal chemotherapy. Vascular access procedures such as short-term percutaneously inserted central catheters as well as indwelling port placements are also common. Patients may be profoundly pancytopenic at presentation, with a resultant increased risk of hemorrhage. Depending on the specific procedure, patients may require platelet transfusion to decrease this risk, particularly before neuraxial procedures.

During treatment with chemotherapeutic agents, patients can be immunocompromised and at increased risk of upper respiratory tract or other infections. Chemotherapy agents can cause systemic toxicity. For example, doxorubicin is known to cause both immediate and long-term cardiac toxicity, and bleomycin predisposes patients to developing pulmonary fibrosis, which can worsen with exposure to high concentrations of inspired oxygen. A full review of anesthetic considerations for oncology patients and related chemotherapy toxicities is outside the scope of this review and has been covered in several comprehensive articles.[1,2] If under active treatment, these patients may have associated nausea and vomiting, with implications for airway management and hydration status. Specific concerns for patients with an anterior mediastinal mass are reviewed elsewhere in this article.

Conjoined Twins

A unique situation encountered at large pediatric tertiary care centers is conjoined twins. The prevalence is estimated to range from 1 in 50,000 to 1 in 100,000 births.[3]

Most conjoined twins require anesthesia for medical imaging studies before separation. The general principles of anesthesia for conjoined twins has been discussed in several comprehensive reviews.[4,5] The type of conjoining determines the specific studies needed, because the possible areas of fusion are predictable in each type. Interventional procedures such as diagnostic angiography may be necessary to determine complex, and shared, vascular components. Almost every organ system will need to be investigated thoroughly, taking into consideration shared organs and body parts. Shared organs need to be evaluated, because cross-circulation is always present to varying degrees. Mixing of blood is an issue in shared organs as well as direct intervascular communications between twins. The extent of the shared organs and vasculature and the effect on the pharmacokinetics and pharmacodynamics of a drug, as well as fluid and blood administration, need to be appreciated and ideally determined before separation.[4] Additionally, problems with intravenous access issues should be anticipated and addressed before the day of separation. Plans should be made to have large-bore central venous access catheters placed in each twin by either a surgeon or interventional radiologist before the day of separation.

PROCEDURE-SPECIFIC CONSIDERATIONS
Interventional Radiology

In adults, many IR procedures are successfully completed either under local anesthesia or with nurse-assisted minimal to moderate sedation. In contrast, pediatric patients often require deep sedation or general anesthesia. As noted, consideration should be given to the age, maturity, and comorbidities of the patient, as well as the consequences of patient movement, as well as the duration, level of stimulation, and likelihood of complications of the particular procedure. IR procedures can be broadly categorized as vascular or nonvascular. Exposure of patients and personnel to radiation and reactions to intravenous radiocontrast media (RCM) in the IR suite are also discussed.

Nonvascular Procedures

Nonvascular procedures performed in the IR suite include gastrostomy and gastrojejunostomy tube placement, image-guided drainage of fluid collections, biopsies of masses and vital organs, lumbar puncture, and esophageal dilation.

Placement of Drainage Catheters

Drainage catheters can be used for the diagnosis and treatment of fluid collections. Depending on the location, ultrasound imaging can be used to assist with placement and fluoroscopic examination can be used for confirmation. Alternatively, drainage procedures can be accomplished with computed tomography (CT) guidance. The location of the collection, patient positioning, and the patient's comorbidities determine whether these procedures can be managed with either moderate to deep sedation or general anesthesia. An additional consideration is that, during CT guidance or fluoroscopy, patient movement means additional radiation exposure when repeated imaging sequences are obtained. Simple fluid collections can be managed with smaller 5- to 8-Fr catheters, whereas complex collections often need larger 12- to 14-Fr catheters for successful drainage.[6] At our institution, when CT guidance is deemed necessary, the interventional procedure is performed in the CT scanner; this measure often poses both scheduling and logistical challenges in managing limited anesthesia resources.

Biopsies

Biopsies in pediatric patients are performed to obtain tissue for diagnosis of masses, and inflammatory or fibrotic processes, and to monitor transplant recipients for signs of rejection. Anesthetic management should consider patient positioning, comorbidities, and the location of the tissue to be sampled. For biopsies near vascular structures or of solid organs, an active type and screen is recommended because, although hemorrhage is rare, it can be significant.[7]

Several imaging modalities have been used successfully. CT guidance can be advantageous for targets that are deep and small. For larger and more superficial structures, ultrasound examination also allows real-time imaging without radiation exposure. Fluoroscopy can be useful for lung or bone lesions. Liver biopsies can be performed with ultrasound imaging, which helps to avoid vascular structures. In patients with significant liver disease resulting in coagulopathy and ascites, biopsies can be obtained through a transjugular approach.[6] Renal biopsies can also be obtained with ultrasound guidance. For native kidneys, patients may be positioned lateral or prone. Transplanted kidneys in the iliac fossa are accessed with the patient supine. Complications from solid organ biopsies include hemorrhage and organ-specific issues. Liver biopsies can cause bile sepsis and hypotension in addition to bleeding complications.[8] Renal biopsies can cause arteriovenous fistula and hematuria, as well as hematomas.[8] Most perinephric hematomas are managed conservatively.[6] Lung biopsies can lead to pneumothorax and hemoptysis. At our institution, we monitor for pneumothorax with fluoroscopy at the conclusion of the biopsy followed by a portable chest radiographs during the recovery period.

Biopsy in Patients with an Anterior Mediastinal Mass

Patients with anterior mediastinal oncologic masses require special caution on the part of the anesthesiologist. For such patients, the dangers of anesthetic agents and positive pressure ventilation and their potential to precipitate hemodynamic or respiratory collapse are well known.[9,10] In particular, pediatric oncology patients with non-Hodgkin lymphoma, Hodgkin lymphoma, or acute lymphocytic leukemia should be evaluated carefully because these oncologic processes can be rapidly enlarging.[11,12]

Patients with anterior mediastinal lesions may have cardiovascular and respiratory effects from the compression of the mass on vital anterior mediastinal structures. The mass can impinge on and compress the trachea, bronchi, superior vena cava, pulmonary arteries, or heart.[9] Patients may also have a pericardial effusion associated with their underlying disease. Obstruction caused by the mass can severely decrease cardiac output, decrease venous return, and cause external compression of the airways.[10] Difficulty swallowing can result from esophageal compression or recurrent laryngeal nerve impingement.

The history and physical examination should focus on elucidating which structures are involved and the severity of symptoms. This focus can help to predict the likelihood of problems on induction of anesthesia and assist in planning the procedural and anesthetic technique, including how to manage adverse intraoperative events. It is important to elicit a history of dyspnea, orthopnea, or stridor and whether these symptoms worsen with position changes. These symptoms may correlate with tracheal or bronchial compression and the likelihood of perioperative complications.[9,13] If a specific position helps to relieve symptoms, the anesthesiologist should use this "rescue position" if there are difficulties with ventilation during the case.[9] Symptoms of superior vena cava syndrome can include plethora of the head and neck, distended superficial veins, and jugular venous distension. Isolated jugular venous distension could indicate tamponade physiology owing to a pericardial effusion rather than superior vena cava syndrome.[9] A paradoxic increase in blood pressure as a patient goes from standing to supine could be a sign of obstruction to right ventricular filling or ejection.[9]

Data specific to the evaluation of anterior mediastinal masses in pediatric patients are generally retrospective and observational in nature. These data are limited by the fact that anesthetic and procedural techniques were likely modified to decrease risk in patients thought to have a higher likelihood of complications. A retrospective review of 118 pediatric patients with oncologic mediastinal masses found that several symptoms and radiologic findings were associated with anesthesia-related complications. These included orthopnea, upper body edema, great vessel compression, and main stem bronchus compression.[13] Another retrospective study of 54 pediatric patients with mediastinal malignancy and a widened mediastinum on chest radiograph found that only stridor was significantly associated with anesthetic complications. However, 33% of these patients received steroids before their anesthetic because they were deemed to be at high risk for complications.[14]

Radiologic studies can also be used for risk stratification. A retrospective review of 46 pediatric patients with anterior mediastinal masses found that, although the majority of patients who had cardiovascular or respiratory symptoms also had findings of cardiorespiratory compression on radiologic imaging, 4 were asymptomatic even though they had imaging evidence of compression.[15] This underscores the importance of thoroughly assessing both patient symptoms and imaging studies. Chest radiographs can be used to calculate a mediastinal mass ratio, which is the maximum width of the mediastinal mass/maximum thoracic width (in centimeters).[14] A study of 51 patients with non-Hodgkin lymphoma or Hodgkin lymphoma found an association between severity of respiratory symptoms and a higher mediastinal mass ratio. Of patients with stridor, all had an mediastinal mass ratio of 45% or higher.[16] Other studies have not found this clear association, or it has not attained statistical significance.[13,14] In the research setting, there is some variability in specific technique used to calculate the tracheal compression seen on CT scan. CT scans can also yield information on main stem bronchus compression. Hack and colleagues[14] reported that perioperative respiratory complications only occurred in patients who either had a tracheal cross-sectional area of less than 30% of normal or less than 70% of normal in those who also had bronchial compression. Anghelescu and colleagues[13] found an association between main stem bronchus compression and anesthetic complications, but the association between tracheal compression and complications did not attain statistical significance. Nonetheless, these findings should be viewed in light of their retrospective nature, relatively small sample size, and likely changes in management for those patients deemed to be at high risk of perioperative events. Some authors recommend avoiding general anesthesia if the tracheal cross-sectional area is less than 50% predicted.[12]

Our institutional protocol for patients with anterior mediastinal masses who present for a diagnostic biopsy is to avoid general anesthesia if possible. For patients with Hodgkin lymphoma or non-Hodgkin lymphoma, the diagnosis can often be made with bone marrow aspirate or biopsy. For other patients, modifying the biopsy target may avoid the need for general anesthesia. For example, a superficial lymph node biopsy may provide sufficient tissue to establish a diagnosis. For patients with severe respiratory symptoms in whom sedation or general anesthesia could be life threatening, we recommend treatment with steroids, chemotherapy, or radiation before biopsy, even though these treatments can make the biopsy results less accurate.[15] For preoperative evaluation of these patients, we recommend chest radiographs with anteroposterior and lateral views, chest CT scanning to evaluate tracheal and bronchial compression, and an echocardiogram to evaluate the inflow and outflow tracts as well as for pericardial effusion.

In situations when sedation or general anesthesia is deemed necessary, anesthetic planning is based on avoiding respiratory and cardiovascular obstruction. Loss of muscle tone and lack of spontaneous ventilation can both cause increased airway compression and precipitate difficulty with ventilation. Most authors recommend maintenance of spontaneous ventilation.[11,15] However, backup plans to treat respiratory compromise or loss of the airway should be available. The supine position can exacerbate cardiovascular and respiratory compromise.[11,12]

Knowing the location of the tracheal or bronchial compression can assist in preoperative planning. For tracheal masses, it may be possible to place an endotracheal tube past the obstruction, possibly with the aid of a rigid bronchoscope and assistance from otolaryngology colleagues. In patients with more distal bronchial compression, intubation or tracheostomy may not relieve the obstruction.[10] However, it may be possible to use single-lung ventilation if the mass is confined to one side. If there is concurrent pulmonary artery compression, it is important to assess for possible ventilation and perfusion mismatching.[9] Moving the patient to their "rescue position" can be used to relieve either respiratory or cardiovascular obstruction.[9,11] Superior vena cava syndrome may be a cause of obstruction to venous return from the upper extremities. If superior vena cava syndrome is suspected, lower extremity intravascular access should be established. Availability of cardiopulmonary bypass and personnel must be set up well in advance for this to be feasible as a rescue strategy in an emergency. In adults, some authors suggest awake preparations for cardiopulmonary bypass,[10] whereas others note that even with advanced preparation there would likely be neurologic injury in the setting of hypoxia.[9] There are few data or recommendations in pediatric patients.

Vascular Procedures

Procedure duration can vary widely, from short vascular access placement to endovascular embolizations lasting more than 8 hours. Meticulous attention to positioning is necessary to prevent patient injuries, because access to the patient may be nearly impossible during the case.

Percutaneously Inserted Central Catheter Lines, Central Venous Catheters, and Indwelling Ports

Percutaneously inserted central catheters provide central venous access for a period of several weeks. They are generally placed above the elbow for ease of movement, preferentially in the basilic vein owing to lower complication risks.[17] Longer term access can be achieved with tunneled central venous catheters. These catheters have a cuff in the tunneled portion that acts as a barrier to infection and helps to prevent accidental dislodgement. However, this cuff makes subsequent line removal more difficult than percutaneously inserted central line removal. Implantable venous ports lack direct cutaneous access and are used for patients who require periodic intravascular access.[18] Of note, patients who have implantable ports and cuffed catheters usually require an anesthetic to have these devices removed at the completion of their treatment protocol. Additionally, these lines may need to be replaced or manipulated in IR if they malfunction before completion of the patient's treatment, thereby necessitating an additional anesthetic.

Vascular Imaging Procedures

Although noninvasive CT and magnetic resonance angiography have replaced diagnostic angiography in many circumstances, conventional angiography still allows better evaluation of small vessels and complex lesions.[18] Cerebral angiogram can be used to aid in the evaluation of patients with a history of stroke or hemorrhage, including diagnosis of the underlying etiology, such as Moyamoya disease.[19] General anesthesia with an endotracheal tube is usually required for cerebral angiograms because it facilitates patient immobility, apnea, and either normocarbia or hypercarbia. Hypercarbia causes dilation of the cerebral blood vessels and can thus facilitate catheter movement by the interventionalist. If there is vasospasm or difficulty maneuvering the catheter through small vessels, the interventional radiologist may administer small doses of nitroglycerin through the catheter. Local doses of nitroglycerin do not typically cause systemic hypotension.[20] Patients must remain supine and lie flat for several hours after removal of the femoral arterial sheath at the conclusion of the angiogram. Beyond parental assistance with behavioral modification, patients may require some level of sedation. In appropriate patients, deep extubation can help to decrease movement and assist with maintaining hemostasis.[19] Dexmedetomidine can be useful because it preserves respiratory drive while providing sedation and anxiolysis.

Patients with Moyamoya disease frequently need cerebral angiograms for diagnosis and preoperative planning. Patients may be on antiplatelet agents and calcium channel blockers, and those with seizures may be on antiepileptics preoperatively.[21] These patients require special precautions to prevent transient ischemic attacks or strokes during the procedure through maintenance of a favorable cerebral oxygen supply to oxygen demand ratio and preservation of cerebral perfusion pressure. Areas affected by the disease depend on blood pressure for perfusion owing to impaired autoregulation.[21] Overall management principles include good hydration before induction to minimize hypotension as well as maintenance of normocarbia. Hypocarbia can lead to further narrowing of cerebral blood vessels with resultant ischemia. Hypercarbia in these patients may cause vasodilation of normal blood vessels while diseased vessels do not dilate, which can lead to decreased flow to areas already prone to ischemia.[21] In our institution, these patients receive an intravenous line preoperatively and a fluid bolus of 20 mL/kg normal saline or lactated Ringer's. Because crying can cause hypocarbia, patients are given a premedication, typically midazolam, before intravenous line placement. The goal blood pressure is at, or above, baseline with a mean arterial pressure that is at least the 50th percentile for their age. During induction, a sympathetic response to laryngoscopy can cause an increase in the cerebral metabolic rate of oxygen consumption and is undesirable. Our institutional protocol recommends a 5 μg/kg fentanyl bolus during induction to blunt this sympathetic response while preserving blood pressure. An induction with either intravenous anesthetics or volatile agents can be used safely, as long as it is titrated according to the hemodynamic and cerebrovascular principles noted, with the goal of maintaining normocarbia. Some authors recommend avoiding ketamine owing to its effect on increasing cerebral metabolic rate.[21]

Glucagon is sometimes used to improve abdominal or pelvic angiographic image quality. Glucagon can cause hyperglycemia, tachycardia, hypertension, and postprocedure hypotonia and vomiting. Rapid administration has been associated with anaphylaxis.[20,22]

Vascular Malformations

Vascular malformations are congenital, abnormal connections between veins, lymphatics, and arterial blood vessels. Although present at birth, they may grow in response to hormones or other stimuli and present later in life. Enlargement over time can necessitate treatment for even asymptomatic malformations.[20] Vascular malformations are generally classified as high flow or low flow.

High-flow lesions include arteriovenous fistulas, arteriovenous malformations, and even large hemangiomas. Patients can develop high-output cardiac failure as infants, or seizures, strokes, and hydrocephalus at older ages. Pulmonary edema can further complicate the management of these patients.[22]

Vein of Galen malformation is a type of arteriovenous fistula that is formed prenatally and can often be diagnosed on prenatal ultrasound examination. These malformations can also present in the postnatal period when high flow through the arteriovenous shunt causes other signs and symptoms. These symptoms include high-output cardiac failure, hydrocephalus, seizures and, rarely, intracerebral hemorrhage. On examination, patients may have prominent scalp and facial veins, an audible scalp bruit, and signs of cardiac failure or hydrocephalus. Patient evaluation should include assessment of their risk for elevated intracranial pressure and cardiac failure. This technically challenging transarterial procedure consists of placements of coils or glue in the malformation to slow blood flow.[18]

Low-flow lesions are composed of venous and lymphatic vessels. These malformations can increase in size over time and become symptomatic. Symptoms result from venous distention and stasis, mass effect, and, rarely, hemorrhage.[18] Endovascular sclerotherapy and embolization can decrease the size of these lesions, but multiple treatments are often necessary.[23] For complex malformations, general anesthesia allows patients to remain completely motionless during this lengthy procedure. Additionally, sclerosing agents cause significant pain, both during the procedure and afterward. Procedure-related swelling can also contribute to patient discomfort.

Agents commonly used for sclerotherapy of venous malformations include sodium tetradecyl sulfate (3%, STS) and ethanol (97%–99%), with other agents used less frequently. Gulsen and colleagues[24] reported the use of polidocanol (2%) in a small study of 19 pediatric patients with venous malformations with similar success rates compared with ethanol. Ethanol and STS cause injury to the vascular endothelium, leading to thrombosis. Ethanol causes denaturation of blood proteins and local hemolysis, which can lead to hemoglobinuria. In a retrospective study of 475 patients who received STS or ethanol for sclerotherapy, Barranco-Pons and colleagues[25] found that 34% developed transient hemoglobinuria, with 57% of patients who had hemoglobinuria also developing transient oliguria. All patients were given crystalloid to replace their fluid deficit and continued on twice maintenance fluid during the procedure. Patients with hemoglobinuria were changed to 5% dextrose in water with 75 mEq/L sodium bicarbonate at twice the maintenance rate. All cases of hemoglobinuria and oliguria resolved. Furosemide can be added to this treatment regimen.[22] Ethanol intoxication is a dose-dependent complication, with behavioral changes and increased risk of respiratory depression. Patients receiving more than 0.75 mL/kg of ethanol are at greater risk.[26] The most severe, but rare, complication is cardiovascular collapse, although the mechanism is unclear. Bradycardia and hypoxemia can portend impending cardiovascular collapse.[20] Migration of thromboembolisms to the lungs can also cause hypoxemia.[20] Ethanol and opiates can cause synergistic respiratory depression.[20]

Patients with vascular malformations are at risk of coagulopathy from several distinct etiologies. Large hemangiomas, tufted angiomas, and hemangioendotheliomas can trap platelets and cause a consumptive thrombocytopenia and depletion of coagulation factors, known at Kasabach-Merritt syndrome.[20,27] Patients with venous malformations can have a consumptive coagulopathy that is similar to disseminated intravascular coagulation and benefit from optimization in consultation with hematology before the procedure. Treatment-related coagulopathy may also occur. After extensive embolization procedures, patients can develop a disseminated intravascular coagulation–like coagulation disturbance known as systemic intravascular coagulopathy.[20] Ethanol and STS are associated with coagulation abnormalities as well.[28]

Approximately 40% of venous malformations occur in the head and neck.[18] These patients require particular attention to the airway, because there can be engorgement of vessels. Swelling can develop or worsen over the course of the procedure, leading to potential airway obstruction postoperatively. The decision to extubate at the end of the procedure should also take into account that edema can continue to worsen after the procedure.[7,20]

Neuroendovascular Tumor Embolization

Preoperative surgical embolization of vascular neoplasms can help to decrease surgical bleeding. The cumulative risk of undergoing embolization followed by surgery versus surgery alone can help to guide the decision to use this treatment modality. General anesthesia with an endotracheal tube is required for immobilization and control of ventilation. Patients with tumors near the airway should be evaluated for potential obstruction. Highly vascular tumors typically have multiple feeding arteries and some of these also supply vital areas, including cerebral, spinal, and retinal tissues. It is important to avoid embolization of these arteries. Inadvertent embolization of arteries that provide dual supply to the tumor and vital tissues with subsequent infarction of vital tissue is a possible complication.[29] The anesthesiologist in these cases should know that it is important to avoid hypercapnia, because it can induce cerebral vasodilation and cause an increased flow of embolic microparticles beyond the area of intended treatment with potential embolization of arteries supplying nontumoral tissue.[29]

Ophthalmic Artery Chemosurgery

Retinoblastoma is the most common intraocular malignancy in childhood.[30] Although cryotherapy and laser therapy can be used for smaller tumors, the vast majority of patients have tumors that are too large for these modalities at diagnosis.[31] Therapies for larger tumors such as radiation and enucleation have notable drawbacks. These include facial disfigurement and later eye complications owing to radiation therapy and blindness after enucleation. Owing to these issues, systemic chemotherapy has been used with improved overall success rates, but patients experience the side effects of systemically administered chemotherapeutic agents. Administration of chemotherapy via intraarterial injection into the ophthalmic artery is a technique designed to minimize systemic effects of chemotherapy while still providing effective treatment for larger tumors.[30,31] There is some variability in the specific institutional protocols for this procedure; however, all require general anesthesia with an endotracheal tube, neuromuscular blocking drugs, and preparation for possible adverse respiratory and cardiovascular events during the procedure. Scharoun and coauthors[31] describe their institutional practice in a recent review article as follows. First, the ipsilateral nare is topicalized with a vasoconstrictor such as oxymetazoline (0.05%) to decrease flow through potential connections between the ophthalmic artery and the external carotid system, which could bypass the intended delivery of chemotherapeutic agents to the tumor via the central retinal artery. Vascular access is obtained via the femoral artery and the patient is given heparin. A microcatheter is then advanced into the orifice of the ophthalmic artery via the internal carotid artery. After ensuring that the catheter is in the correct position, chemotherapeutic agents such as melphalan, topotecan, and carboplatin are administered over a period of approximately 30 minutes. All patients are given antiemetics and extubated in a manner to minimize coughing, which may include deep extubation if this is otherwise clinically appropriate. Dexmedetomidine given during emergence can facilitate compliance with lying flat after the procedure. Patients are required to remain supine and flat for 5 hours to prevent hematoma formation at the femoral access site.[31] These patients are at increased risk of postprocedure nausea and vomiting, which is particularly undesirable after removal of femoral arterial access.[19] Local complications at the femoral access site have been reported; strokes and hemorrhage are theoretically possible, but have not been reported.[30] Earlier versions of this procedure involved using a balloon to occlude distal flow at the branch point of the ophthalmic artery before infusion of chemotherapy; catheterization of the ophthalmic artery was adopted as a later modification. In the event of an inability to cannulate the ophthalmic artery, the earlier technique of distal balloon occlusion can be used.[30]

Anesthesiologists involved in the care of patients undergoing intraarterial chemotherapy injection must be prepared to treat several potential adverse events that may occur during treatment. The major respiratory and cardiovascular complications associated with the procedure involve mechanisms that are not as yet fully understood although several reflexes have been proposed as possible causes.[31] During catheterization of the internal carotid artery or ophthalmic artery, patients can show abrupt decreases in pulmonary compliance. Decreases in oxygen saturation can also occur. This complication typically manifests as a sudden decrease in tidal volumes, higher peak airway pressures, and oxygen desaturation that are not accompanied by wheezing. The capnogram generally does not show an obstructive pattern and preemptive treatment with albuterol or steroids has not clinically prevented the issue.[31] In a retrospective review of 468 cases, Kato and colleagues[32] found that 29% of cases had an event characterized by a decrease in pulmonary compliance of 40% or greater. In addition to asking the neuroradiologist to stop catheter manipulation and supporting oxygenation with 100% inspired fraction of oxygen, treatment is with epinephrine boluses of 0.5 to 1.0 µg/kg.[31] Hemodynamic instability with bradycardia and hypotension has also been described. Some authors suggest that hypotension and bradycardia tend to occur after the onset of respiratory changes.[33] Other authors posit that the use of epinephrine to treat decreased pulmonary compliance may prevent subsequent bradycardia and hypotension.[31]

Exposure to Radiation

The patients and staff in the pediatric IR suite are at risk for long-term complications owing to radiation exposure. Pediatric patients have several factors that place them at greater risk of developing radiation-induced malignancies than adults. During growth, cells have a higher mitotic rate and are more susceptible to DNA damage. Because children have more years of life ahead of them than adults, there is more time for malignancies to develop. The accumulated radiation dose for patients with chronic conditions requiring repeated treatments can approach that known to be associated with an increased cancer risk. Additionally, children with certain syndromes may be less able to repair radiation-induced DNA damage and thus more likely to develop malignancies.[34] Efforts to limit radiation exposure include limiting the number of studies by substituting ultrasound examination and MRI scans when possible, and following pediatric-specific dose limiting protocols. Strategies used during angiography can include removing the grid in infants, decreasing the space between the image receptor and the patient, optimizing the distance between the patient and the radiation source, and shielding the patient with lead.[6] Other dose reduction strategies include the use of pulsed fluoroscopy, the use of saved angiographic runs as a vessel map that can be reused, and coning and positioning patients without using fluoroscopy.[35]

Anesthesiologists who are exposed to radiation are at risk for the long-term development of malignancies and cataracts. Scatter can cause the anesthesiologist at the head of the bed to have higher radiation exposure than the interventional radiologist.[19] Recommended steps to minimize exposure include wearing wraparound lead aprons and protective leaded glasses, and placement of a lead shield between the anesthesiologist and the patient. Radiation follows the inverse square law: increased distance from the radiation source decreases the radiation dose. If possible, the anesthesiologist should leave the room during angiography and fluoroscopy runs. Dosimeter badges should be used to monitor cumulative exposure. During lateral fluoroscopy, standing on the same side as the image receptor decreases the dose of radiation owing to scatter.[34]

Adverse Reactions to Radiographic Contrast Media

Anesthesiologists caring for patients in IR should be aware of the potential effects and adverse reactions from intravenous contrast materials. Serious adverse effects are more likely to occur with high osmolality contrast media (1–2 per 1000), but can still occur with low osmolality contrast media (1–2 per 10,000)[36] and nonionic contrast. Reactions to RCM can be separated into immediate and delayed reactions, with immediate reactions occurring within 1 hour of administration.[37] Less severe immediate reactions include nausea, vomiting, or urticaria. Delayed reactions usually present with exanthemas.[37] Other reactions to contrast include anxiety, fever, facial flushing, seizures, and pulmonary edema.[36]

Anaphylactoid reactions to RCM usually occur within 5 minutes of administration[37] up to the first hour,[19] but have been reported several hours later.[36] Symptoms can include bronchospasm and cardiovascular instability. We recommend use of the Society for Pediatric Anesthesia PediCrisis algorithm for managing anaphylaxis, which is available online[38] or through a free mobile device application available on iTunes as the Pediatric Critical Events Checklist. Patients at higher risk of adverse reactions to RCM include those with asthma and other atopic disease, and those with a prior history of reactions to RCM.[19,37]

Other effects of RCM relate to its hypertonicity. This effect causes several hemodynamic changes with administration. There may be transient hypotension directly after administration that resolves quickly, followed by a period of increased blood pressure as extravascular fluid moves intravascularly. After about 10 minutes, equilibration occurs. The RCM then causes a diuresis that requires close attention to volume status with respect to increased urine output.[36] For children with cardiovascular instability, these hemodynamic changes may be more clinically significant.

Renal failure owing to RCM has also been reported. Children with preexisting renal disease, cardiovascular disease, diabetes mellitus, hyperuricemia, and dehydration are at greater risk.[36] Children with paraproteinemia are at higher risk for irreversible renal failure, which should be prevented with adequate intravenous hydration.[36]

Finally, attention to dose limits of RCM is important. At our institution, we use nonionic triiodinated iohexol, 300 mg iodine/mL, and limit our doses to 3 mL/kg. Other authors have recommended use of 240 mg iodine/mL of nonionic contrast, with a dose limit of 2 mL/kg.[35] This dose can be easily exceeded in smaller patients and underscores the responsibility of the anesthesiologist to ensure patient immobility during contrast injection to allow adequate studies to be obtained.

SUMMARY

Technologic advances have increased the numbers of pediatric patients undergoing procedures in IR. Indeed, anesthesiologists are increasingly being called on to care for pediatric patients with complex medical issues in the IR suite. The availability of minimally invasive approaches can provide significant patient benefit. Familiarity with the specific patient populations and procedures as well as potential procedure-specific complications can facilitate anesthetic planning and management. However, the non–operating room anesthesia setting with its unfamiliar environment and personnel can pose certain challenges. To provide the best care possible to some of our most medically complicated pediatric patients, preparation has to include close communication with the entire IR team about the patient's comorbidities and the planned procedure.

REFERENCES

1. Latham GJ, Greenberg RS. Anesthetic considerations for the pediatric oncology patient—part 1: a review of antitumor therapy. Paediatr Anaesth 2010;20: 295–304.
2. Latham GJ, Greenberg RS. Anesthetic considerations for the pediatric oncology patient—part 2: systems-based approach to anesthesia. Paediatr Anaesth 2010; 20:396–420.
3. Spitz L, Kiely EM. Conjoined twins. JAMA 2003;289(10):1307–10.
4. Szmuk P, Rabb MF, Curry B, et al. Anaesthetic management of thoracopagus twins with complex cyanotic heart disease for cardiac assessment: special considerations related to ventilation and cross-circulation. Br J Anaesth 2006;96(3): 341–5.
5. Thomas J. Anesthesia for conjoined twins. In: Davis PJ, Cladis FP, Motoyama EK, editors. Smith's anesthesia for infants and children. 8th edition. Philadelphia: Elsevier Mosby; 2011. p. 950–70.
6. Burrill J, Heran MK. Nonvascular pediatric interventional radiology. Can Assoc Radiol J 2012;63:s49–58.
7. Landrigan-Ossar M. Common procedures and strategies for anaesthesia in interventional radiology. Curr Opin Anaesthesiol 2015;28(4):458–63.
8. Norman J. Practical pediatric interventional radiology. Curr Probl Diagn Radiol 2001;30(3):66–86.
9. Blank RS, de Souza D. Anesthetic management of patients with an anterior mediastinal mass: continuing professional development. Can J Anaesth 2011;58: 853–67.
10. Goh MH, Goh YS. Anterior mediastinal mass: an anaesthetic challenge. Anaesthesia 1999;54:670–82.
11. Lerman J. Anterior mediastinal masses in children. Semin Anesth 2007;26: 133–40.
12. Perger L, Lee EY, Shamberger RC. Management of children and adolescents with a critical airway due to compression by an anterior mediastinal mass. J Pediatr Surg 2008;43:1990–7.
13. Anghelescu DL, Burgoyne LL, Liu T, et al. Clinical and diagnostic imaging findings predict anesthetic complications in children presenting with malignant mediastinal masses. Paediatr Anaesth 2007;17:1090–8.
14. Hack HA, Wright NB, Wynn RF. The anaesthetic management of children with anterior mediastinal masses. Anaesthesia 2008;63:837–46.

15. Stricker PA, Gurnaney HG, Litman RS. Anesthetic management of children with an anterior mediastinal mass. J Clin Anesth 2010;22:159–63.
16. King DR, Patrick LE, Ginn-Pease ME, et al. Pulmonary function is compromised in children with mediastinal lymphoma. J Pediatr Surg 1997;32:294–300.
17. Krishnamurthy G, Keller MS. Vascular access in children. Cardiovasc Intervent Radiol 2011;34:14–24.
18. Heran MK, Burill J. Vascular pediatric interventional radiology. Can Assoc Radiol J 2012;63(3):s59–73.
19. Landrigan-Ossar M, McClain CD. Anesthesia for interventional radiology. Paediatr Anaesth 2014;24:698–702.
20. Mason KP. Pediatric procedures in interventional radiology. Int Anesthesiol Clin 2009;47(3):35–43.
21. Parray T, Martin TW, Siddiqui S. Moyamoya disease: a review of the disease and anesthetic management. J Neurosurg Anesthesiol 2011;23(2):100–9.
22. Mason KP. Pediatric anesthesia outside of the operating room. In: Urman RD, Gross WL, Philip BK, editors. Anesthesia outside of the operating room. New York: Oxford University Press; 2011. p. 236–43.
23. Uehara S, Osuga K, Yoneda A, et al. Intralesional sclerotherapy for subcutaneous venous malformations in children. Pediatr Surg Int 2009;25:709–13.
24. Gulsen F, Cantasdemir M, Solak S, et al. Percutaneous sclerotherapy of peripheral venous malformations in pediatric patients. Pediatr Surg Int 2011;27:1283–7.
25. Barranco-Pons R, Burrows PE, Landrigan-Ossar M, et al. Gross hemoglobinuria and oliguria are common transient complications of sclerotherapy for venous malformations: review of 475 procedures. AJR Am J Roentgenol 2012;199:691–4.
26. Mason KP, Michna E, Zurakowski D, et al. Serum ethanol levels in children and adults after ethanol embolization or sclerotherapy for vascular anomalies. Radiology 2000;217:127–32.
27. Elsayes KM, Menias CO, Dillman JR, et al. Vascular malformations and hemangiomatosis syndromes: spectrum of imaging manifestations. AJR Am J Roentgenol 2008;190(5):1291–9.
28. Mason KP, Neufeld EJ, Karian VE, et al. Coagulation abnormalities in pediatric and adult patients after sclerotherapy or embolization of vascular anomalies. AJR Am J Roentgenol 2001;177:1359–63.
29. Abruzzo TA, Heran MKS. Neuroendovascular therapies in pediatric interventional radiology. Tech Vasc Interv Radiol 2011;14(1):50–6.
30. Jarbour P, Chalouhi N, Tjoumakaris S, et al. Pearls and pitfalls of intra-arterial chemotherapy for retinoblastoma. J Neurosurg Pediatr 2012;10:175–81.
31. Scharoun JH, Han JH, Gobin P. Anesthesia for ophthalmic artery chemosurgery. Anesthesiology 2017;126(1):165–72.
32. Kato MA, Green N, O'Connell K, et al. A retrospective analysis of severe intraoperative respiratory compliance changes during ophthalmic arterial chemosurgery for retinoblastoma. Paediatr Anaesth 2015;25:595–602.
33. Phillips TJ, McGuirk SP, Chahal HK, et al. Autonomic cardio-respiratory reflex reactions and superselective ophthalmic arterial chemotherapy for retinoblastoma. Paediatr Anaesth 2013;23:940–5.
34. Sidhu M, Strauss KJ, Connolly B, et al. Radiation safety in pediatric interventional radiology. Tech Vasc Interv Radiol 2010;13:158–66.
35. Lord DJ. The practice of pediatric interventional radiology. Tech Vasc Interv Radiol 2011;14:2–7.

36. Cravero J. Anesthesia outside the operating room. In: Cote CJ, Lerman J, Anderson B, editors. A practice of anesthesia for infants and children. 5th edition. Philadelphia: Elsevier Saunders; 2013. p. 963–79.

37. Brockow K, Ring J. Anaphylaxis to radiographic contrast media. Curr Opin Allergy Clin Immunol 2011;11:326–31.

38. PediCrisis Critical Events Cards. In: Society for Pediatric Anesthesia. 2015. Available at: http://www.pedsanesthesia.org/wp-content/uploads/2015/12/Critical EventsChecklists_12142015.pdf. Accessed January 21, 2017.

Market Evaluation
Finances, Bundled Payments, and Accountable Care Organizations

Shazia Mehmood Siddique, MD[a],*, Shivan J. Mehta, MD, MBA[b]

KEYWORDS

- Health care • Health economics • Bundled payments
- Accountable care organizations • Anesthesia

KEY POINTS

- Increasing health care costs in the United States have resulted in a shift of financial risk to providers for the coordination, quality, and cost of care.
- Although fee-for-service has historically dominated provider payments, newer models, such as pay-for-performance, bundled payments, and accountable care organizations, have the potential for cost savings and quality improvement.
- Regardless of specific policies and payment models, physicians and health systems will need to demonstrate the quality and value of the care they provide.

INTRODUCTION

Health care spending in the United States has been under scrutiny during the past few decades, with rates of spending increasing at a substantial rate. In 2015, national health expenditures grew to $3.2 trillion, accounting for 17.8% of the nation's gross domestic product (**Fig. 1**).[1] In an effort to control costs and improve quality, changes in health care delivery and financing have emerged to improve this fragmented health care system. This trend has resulted in shifting of financial risk to providers for both the quality and cost of care, including the emergence of accountable care organizations (ACOs) and bundled payment models. This article discusses financing and delivery models in the context of procedures and surgeries that happen outside of the traditional operating room setting. It describes the history of health insurance, trends in ambulatory surgery centers, and new payment models that have emerged from the

Disclosure Statement: We have no financial disclosures to report.
[a] Division of Gastroenterology, Perelman School of Medicine, 3400 Civic Center Boulevard–7th Floor Gastroenterology, Philadelphia, PA 19104, USA; [b] Division of Gastroenterology, Perelman School of Medicine, 3400 Civic Center Boulevard–14th Floor Innovation Center, Philadelphia, PA 19104, USA
* Corresponding author.
E-mail address: shazia.siddique@uphs.upenn.edu

Anesthesiology Clin 35 (2017) 715–724
http://dx.doi.org/10.1016/j.anclin.2017.08.005
1932-2275/17/© 2017 Elsevier Inc. All rights reserved.

anesthesiology.theclinics.com

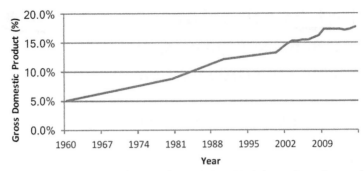

Fig. 1. National health expenditure spending: 1960 to 2015. (*Data from* Centers for Medicare & Medicaid Services. National Health Expenditure Data. NHE Fact Sheet. Available at: https://www.cms.gov/research-statistics-data-and-systems/statistics-trends-and-reports/nationalhealthexpenddata/nhe-fact-sheet.html. Accessed January 13, 2017.)

Affordable Care Act (ACA) and the Medicare Access and Children's Health Insurance Program (CHIP) Reauthorization Act (MACRA).

EVOLUTION OF HEALTH INSURANCE IN THE UNITED STATES

Historically, health insurance in the United States has been primarily through a fee-for-service model, in which providers are paid individually for each service. This started with Blue Cross and Blue Shield plans and Medicare, which paid separately for hospital and physician services. Not surprisingly, this payment model encouraged the delivery of more services because hospitals and physicians were paid for more care. A combination of the fee-for-service payment system, the third-party insurance system, and advances in technology resulted in increasing health care costs.[2]

It became evident by the 1980s that this payment model alone was financially unsustainable. Between 1965 and 1984, there was a 1400% increase in overall Medicare costs, compared with a 242% growth in the consumer price index.[3] Such a large and disproportionate increase placed financial pressure on employers, payers, the government, and patients. Inpatient care, which has historically made up the bulk of health care delivery, has also been the most costly for the Medicare system, with 73% of Medicare expenditures in 1980.[3]

Efforts for cost-containment emerged, leading to Medicare's first major effort to control inpatient spending. Medicare's Inpatient Prospective Payment System (IPPS) was launched in 1983 as an attempt to limit unnecessary utilization of inpatient services because hospitals were historically paid retrospectively based on charges. With IPPS, hospitals were prospectively paid a certain amount based on clinical conditions, or diagnosis-related groups (DRGs). Because hospitals were getting paid the same amount regardless of resource utilization, it encouraged shorter length of stay and a reduction in the increase of inpatient costs, with no measurable impact on quality.[4] These factors contributed to a profound change in economic incentives for hospitals, also encouraging a shift of care to outpatient settings, including ambulatory surgical centers.

As economic incentives changed for hospitals, there was also an evolution in reimbursement for physician services. Historically, medical insurance companies would pay physicians based on a "usual, customary, and reasonable rate." Based on research done by Hsiao and colleagues,[5] there was a transition from charges to the resources needed to provide services, which was called the resource-based relative value scale, which included physician work, practice expense (when performed in a physician office setting), and professional liability costs. Relative value units (RVUs) were used to compare the time and intensity of physician services, and actual payment from Medicare and many commercial payers is based on a conversion factor of RVU.

TRANSITION FROM HOSPITAL-BASED SURGERIES TO AMBULATORY SURGICAL CENTERS

In 1966, Drs David Cohen and John Dillon[6] published a study entitled "Anesthesia for Outpatient Surgery" in JAMA, describing an outpatient surgery pilot program at the University of California, Los Angeles. Motivated by increasing bed shortages, unnecessarily long hospitalizations, and associated high costs for inpatient surgeries, surgeons selected specific operations to occur as outpatient rather than inpatient operations during this pilot. Selection criteria of cases included a maximum predicted postoperative observation time of 3 hours and no evidence of infection. In a sample of 804 subjects, only 4.1% of cases resulted in inpatient admission postoperatively, indicating the feasibility of this pilot. During a 2-year study period (1963–1964), they reported a total estimated savings of $28,000 to patients or insurance companies, and approximately 1000 hospital-days were saved during the study period.

Encouraged by this pilot, Drs. Wallace Reed and John Ford[7,8] opened the first ambulatory surgical center in February 1970, in Phoenix, Arizona, investing in the concept that low-risk surgeries could move away from a complex hospital system and into a lower cost, higher efficiency model. Throughout the 1970s, Drs. Reed and Ford published their findings from their successful Surgicenter to serve as a guide for fellow physicians. They described the provisions necessary to formally establish such a center and to ensure high quality of care for patients, including the regulatory approvals required, the types of equipment stocked, thresholds for deferring surgeries in sicker patients, and postoperative discharge protocols. The initial Surgicenter model continued to primarily use general anesthesia (90% of cases), and the most common operation was diagnostic dilation and curettage, with gynecologic surgeries comprising most cases. They documented the benefits to surgeons, anesthesiologists, and patients, including higher production of surgical cases, ability to stock the latest technology and equipment, and easier facilitation of quality improvement and patient safety efforts.

By the 1980s, health care delivery notably shifted out of the inpatient arena and into outpatient facilities, including physician offices and ambulatory surgical centers. Two major contributors to this shift were newer payment arrangements and technologic and medical advances. Specifically, improved anesthetics and analgesics, alongside newer minimally invasive surgical approaches, allowed for patients to be safely cared for in an outpatient setting, with same-day discharges postoperatively.[9] In 1980, about 3 million operations were done in an ambulatory setting, which grew to 27 million by 1995.[10] Interestingly, during the same period, there was not a notable change in rates of inpatient operations, indicating the expanding utilization of surgeries and procedures in this health care environment. This expansion led to a substantial growth in the health care provider workforce, including anesthesiology. In 1967, there were 8800 anesthesiologists and 13,400 certified registered nurse anesthetists (CRNAs), increasing to 19,000 anesthesiologists and 22,500 CRNAs by 1986. During this 20-year period, the number of anesthesiologists increased by 116%, compared with a 68% increase for CRNAs.[11]

Recent data show that outpatient surgeries made up nearly half of the 19 million surgeries performed in 2012 in community hospitals across 28 states.[12] Many specialties moved a large percentage of their total procedures to ambulatory surgery centers, including gastroenterology and ophthalmology (**Fig. 2**).[13]

However, as the health care system expanded, it also became more fragmented and there were concerns about quality. The fee-for-service model continued to reward the quantity of services rather than the quality of patient care. Problems with care coordination and integration emerged because patients now had multiple sites of care, including urgent care centers, hospitals, outpatient providers, and specialty services.[14] Concern arose that, although the United States had the largest health care spending of all countries, measures of population health and quality lagged behind, such as high infant mortality rates and low life expectancy rates compared with other OECD (Organisation for Economic Cooperation and Development) countries. For example, 2 Institute of Medicine (IOM) reports in 1999 and 2001 addressed patient safety and quality improvement, and issues that required large-scale changes in the health care delivery system.[15,16] Specifically, "To Err is Human" highlighted that tens of thousands Americans die each year from medical errors and, therefore, effectively made patient safety and quality a priority for policymakers. The "Crossing the Quality Chasm" IOM report described broader quality issues and defined 6 aims: care should be safe, effective, patient-centered, timely, efficient, and equitable. The report also recommended that common conditions serve as a starting point for restructuring health care delivery, with an emphasis on decreasing waste, making evidence-based decisions, ensuring transparency, and customizing care according to patient needs and values. These reports shifted the framework for health care delivery, prompting a greater need for multidisciplinary care coordination.

OUTPATIENT CARE COORDINATION

Focus subsequently shifted toward outpatient care coordination and management. In the 1980s and 1990s, the increase of health maintenance organizations emphasized the shift in philosophy toward establishing primary care providers serving as central gatekeepers to specialty services. Although many models allowed for more of an open access model, these health organizations were an attempt at cost containment

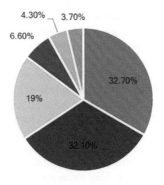

Gastrointestinal ■ Eye ▪ Nervous System ■ Musculoskeletal ▫ Skin ▪ Genitourinary

Fig. 2. Specialty category by volume, CY 2009 ASC claims. ASC, ambulatory surgical center; CY, calendar year. (*Data from* U.S. Department of Health and Human Services. Report to Congress: Medicare Ambulatory Surgical Center Value-Based Purchasing Implementation Plan. Available at: https://www.cms.gov/Medicare/Medicare-Fee-for-Service-Payment/ASCPayment/Downloads/C_ASC_RTC-2011.pdf. Accessed January 26, 2017.)

with a focus on care integration and capitation, or providers taking on more financial risk. The Balanced Budget Act (BBA) of 1997 introduced Part C of Medicare, or Medicare Advantage, which allowed for the administration of Medicare by private insurers, typically though managed care plans. BBA also created the Outpatient Prospective Payment System (OPPS) in 2000 by the Centers for Medicaid and Medicare Services (CMS), which prospectively paid fixed amounts for outpatient facility and skilled nursing facility fees. Throughout the 2000s, several other legislative efforts included revisions to the OPPS, which ultimately established a new payment rate system for medical and surgical services, and created the Hospital Outpatient Quality Reporting (OQR) program.[17] Both the OPPS and OQR encourage financial planning in outpatient care, while meeting quality metrics for outpatients. Some models, such as pay-for-performance, additionally link financial incentives to outcome metrics and have been shown to improve quality of care in some domains.[18]

PATIENT-CENTERED MEDICAL AND SURGICAL HOMES

The concept of a medical home model first emerged in pediatrics in 1967 but began to spread throughout the United States in a variety of disciplines in the late 1980s to 1990s. The patient-centered medical home (PCMH) is a model of primary care management that seeks to meet the health care needs of patients through team-based care, and to improve efficiency through care coordination and a system-based approach to quality and safety.[19]

From an anesthesia perspective, the perioperative surgical home (PSH) is the primary practice model that has been proposed to improve the fragmented and expensive perioperative system. Similar to the medical home, the PSH is a patient-centered and physician-led multidisciplinary team that aims to guide patients throughout the entire surgical experience. A recent review identified key elements that have been applied to this model, including preoperative triage systems with innovation programs for select patients, intraoperative pain and fluid management, integrated scheduling with outpatient and inpatient electronic health record (EHR) systems, and postoperative efforts such as early mobilization with coordination of rehabilitation services and improved patient and caretaker education on perioperative pain and postdischarge care.[20] The concept of medical and surgical homes holds promise for cost reduction and quality improvement within health care.

BUNDLED PAYMENTS

The ACA, enacted in 2010, included the development of the Center for Medicare and Medicaid Innovation (CMMI), which aimed to test innovative payment and delivery models that could reduce costs while maintaining or improving health care quality. CMMI launched the Bundled Payments for Care Improvement (BPCI) initiative in 2013. The concept of bundled payments holds hospitals accountable for all care during the hospital stay, as well as the 90-day period after discharge. Therefore, bundled payments simply refer to the grouping of different medical services across a prespecified episode of care. BPCI includes 4 broadly defined models of care that link payments for multiple services during a defined episode of care, as specified by 48 different DRGs (**Table 1**).[21]

Although the expression bundled payments is a newer terminology, the concept is similar to the original 1983 Medicare IPPS, which is evident in Model 1, as well as the OPPS, as previously described. Models 2 and 3 are retrospective with different definitions of episodes of care, whereas Model 4 is a prospective payment for an inpatient admission. Also, bundled payments have been shown to have a beneficial impact in

Table 1
Bundled payment models

	Model 1	Model 2	Model 3	Model 4
Episode	All DRGs: all acute patients	Selected DRGs: hospital plus postacute period	Selected DRGs; postacute period only	Selected DRGs hospital plus readmissions
Services included	All Part A services paid as part of the DRG payment	All nonhospice Part A and B services during the initial inpatient stay, postacute period, and readmissions	All nonhospice Part A and B services during the postacute period and readmissions	All nonhospice Part A and B services (eg, hospital and physician) during initial inpatient stay and readmissions
Payment	Retrospective	Retrospective	Retrospective	Prospective

From Centers for Medicare & Medicaid Services. Bundled Payments for Care Improvement Initiative (BPCI). Available at: https://www.cms.gov/Newsroom/MediaReleaseDatabase/Fact-sheets/2016-Fact-sheets-items/2016-04-18.html. Accessed January 18 2017; with permission.

the private sector, before BPCI creation. For example, among the most well-known performance-based bundled payments is the Prometheus payment model, developed in 2006.[22] This model assigns evidence-based case reimbursement rates (ECRs) to common conditions such as diabetes and heart failure, as well as common procedures such as joint replacements. A single ECR covers all inpatient and outpatient care associated with a given condition, but these episodes do not necessarily need to be anchored by an inpatient stay; they can relate to a disease condition or outpatient procedure. The Blue Cross and Blue Shield of North Carolina knee replacement bundled-payment includes the presurgical period of 30 days before hospitalization, the surgery, and most follow-up care within 180 days postdischarge, and saved about 8% to 10% on average per-episode cost in a 1-year pilot.[23]

ACCOUNTABLE CARE ORGANIZATIONS

ACOs are groups of hospitals, physicians, and other health care providers who voluntarily work together to improve the value of care for a defined population. The ultimate goal is to ensure patients receive care in a timely fashion while avoiding unnecessary duplication of services and medical errors.[24] The push toward ACOs has come from payers' goal to emphasize the role of primary care provider in care coordination, with a component of payment directly to the quality of care provided. In ACOs, providers take on more risk along the spectrum of provider payment models (**Fig. 3**).

The ACA established the Medicare Shared Savings Program, intended to encourage the development of ACOs in Medicare. Under this program, a Medicare ACO is formed by a group of providers and suppliers of services, such as hospitals and physicians. Eligibility requirements include a minimum of 5000 Medicare fee-for-service beneficiaries, the establishment of an ACO governing body that is responsible for routine self-assessment, monitoring, and quality of care reporting, and a commitment of at least 3 years in the program.[25] If these requirements are met, an ACO application will be reviewed by the Shared Savings Program. Under this program, CMS will initially continue to pay providers and suppliers using the fee-for-service model. Then, using a financial benchmark based on historical expenditures for beneficiaries assigned to that ACO, CMS will retrospectively determine if an ACO will receive shared savings or

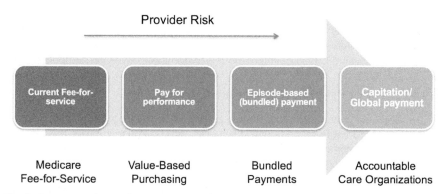

Fig. 3. Spectrum of provider payment models.

owes money due to losses. This amount is also tied to performance on 34 quality metrics, which include measures such as patient survey data via Consumer Assessment of Health Care Providers and Systems, risk-standardized readmission rates, and certain preventive care such as colorectal cancer screening.

The Pioneer ACO model was subsequently launched in 2012, with greater potential savings or losses, focused on organizations that already have experience with care coordination.[26] Between 2012 and 2013, Pioneer ACOs generated approximately $183 million in savings to the Medicare program, compared with the relative projected spending levels, while improving mean quality scores from 70.8% to 84.0%.[26] Although initial reviews of ACOs are overall promising, there have been some concerns. One-third of Pioneer ACOs did not generate lower expenditure growth relative to their comparison populations during the first 2 years and 2 ACOs generated significantly higher expenditure growth during their second year. However, multiple factors may contribute, including variation in time necessary for an ACO to redesign care delivery and adverse selection of high-cost patients. Further research is needed to determine how ACOs in different markets will function, and CMS is currently working to redesign certain elements, such as newer benchmarking methodologies, through their Next Generation ACO model, which opened for application in December 2016.[27] The Next Generation ACO model allows providers to assume higher levels of financial risk and reward, alongside tools to support patient engagement and care management.

THE MEDICARE ACCESS AND CHILDREN'S HEALTH INSURANCE PROGRAM REAUTHORIZATION ACT

In 2015, MACRA became law with bipartisan support, replacing the sustainable growth rate (SGR) for physician reimbursement.[28] The prior SGR was part of BBA in 1997 as a way to control costs related to physician reimbursement from Medicare. However, temporary measures to override the SGR formula had dominated public policy discussions due to payment cliffs that required legislation to override.

Through MACRA, health care professionals are provided with stable fees for 5 years. The Quality Payment Program was launched and included 2 tracks for providers to choose from: the advanced alternative payment models (APMs) or the merit-based incentive payment system (MIPS). The APMs include ACOs, medical homes, and bundled payment arrangements, among others. In terms of MIPS, the plan is to replace and consolidate 3 current existing payment programs: the Physician Quality Reporting System, the meaningful use of EHRs, and the value-based payment modifier. In 2019, providers who participated in MIPS and submitted 2017 data can earn a positive MIPS payment adjustment. Participants in an advanced APM in 2017 may earn a 5% incentive payment in 2019. These provisions within MACRA pave the way for value-based payment models to dominate physician reimbursement.

PROLIFERATION OF NEW PAYMENT MODELS

In 2016, CMS launched the first mandatory postacute bundled payment, the Comprehensive Care for Joint Replacement (CJR) model, which aims to improve the value of care for Medicare beneficiaries undergoing hip and knee replacement surgery. Similar to the previously described bundled payment models, the episode includes an inpatient stay and a 90-day postdischarge period. The CJR model requires participation from IPPS hospitals in 67 metropolitan areas throughout the country, which will be accountable for the cost and quality of care during the episode.[29] This model set a strong precedent for future financial models tied to episodes of care and is an indication of the shift toward value-based payments.

Not only has CMS developed the models described, state Medicaid and commercial insurance companies have also adopted similar models, which reflect payer goals of providing higher quality, lower cost care. Some bundled payment models have naturally followed into the private insurance setting. In other instances, CMS has engaged with multiple other payers for their proposed models, including in an all-payer payment reform initiative in Maryland.[30] The Department of Health and Human Services has set target goals to have 90% of all Medicare fee-for-service payments tied to quality or value by 2018 and, more specifically, 50% of all Medicare payments through alternative payment models by the end of 2018.[31] The passage of MACRA proves also that there is strong bipartisan support to shift toward value-based payment in the current health care system with its increasing costs.

FUTURE DIRECTIONS

Despite uncertainty about the ACA, change in payment and delivery models have actually been evolving over decades. This has been a response to the consistent increasing cost of care, and questions about quality and value. The ACA has accelerated new payment models, particularly in Medicare through the formation of CMMI. Many of these models, such as bundled payments, PCMH, and some forms of ACOs have been proliferating in the commercial insurance market because these payers have similar concerns about cost and quality. Additionally, many of the pay-for-performance mechanisms are independent of ACA. Finally, independent of politics, the economy and health care system will continue to be tasked with finding ways to reduce the increase in health care costs while maintaining quality and access. As with all other specialties and clinical settings, nonoperative anesthesia will have to demonstrate the quality and value of care provided to payers and patients. This includes measuring the quality and outcomes of care, and identifying ways to better coordinate care and reduce variations of care to minimize unnecessary utilization.

REFERENCES

1. Centers for Medicare & Medicaid Services. National Health Expenditure Data Fact Sheet. 2016. Available at: https://www.cms.gov/research-statistics-data-and-systems/statistics-trends-and-reports/nationalhealthexpenddata/nhe-fact-sheet.html. Accessed January 13, 2017.

2. Feinglass J, Holloway JJ. The Initial impact of the medicare prospective payment system on US health care: a review of the literature. Med Care Rev 1991;48(1): 91–115.
3. Freeland M, Schendler C. Health spending in the 1980s: integration of clinical practice patterns with management. Health Care Financ Rev 1984;3:1–68.
4. Coulam RF, Gaumer GL. Medicare's prospective payment system: a critical appraisal. Health Care Financ Rev 1992;1991:45–77.
5. Hsiao WC, Braun P, Yntema D, et al. Estimating physicians' work for a resource-based relative value scale. N Engl J Med 1988;319:835–41.
6. Cohen DD, Dillon JB. Anesthesia for outpatient surgery. JAMA 1966;196(13): 98–100.
7. Ford JL, Reed WA. The surgicenter. An innovation in the delivery and cost of medical care. Ariz Med 1969;26(10):801–14.
8. Reed WA, Ford JL. The surgicenter: an ambulatory surgical facility. Clin Obstet Gynecol 1974;17(3):217–30.
9. Kozak LJ, McCarthy E, Pokras R. Changing patterns of surgical care in the United States: 1980-1985. Health Care Financ Rev 1999;21(1).
10. Kozak LJ, Owings MF. Ambulatory and inpatient procedures in the United States, 1995. Vital Health Stat 13 1998;135:1–116.
11. Rosenbach ML, Cromwell J. A profile of anesthesia practice patterns. Health Aff 1988;7(4):118–31.
12. Inpatient vs. Outpatient Surgeries in U.S. Hospitals. Healthcare Cost and Utilization Project (HCUP). Agency for Healthcare Research and Quality, Rockville, MD. 2015. Available at: www.hcup-us.ahrq.gov/reports/infographics/inpt_outpt.jsp. Accessed January 27, 2017.
13. Centers for Medicare and Medicaid Services. Ambulatory Surgery Centers. 2011. Available at: https://www.cms.gov/Medicare/Medicare-Fee-for-Service-Payment/ASCPayment/Downloads/C_ASC_RTC-2011.pdf. Accessed on January 26, 2017.
14. Fraser I. Ambulatory care and healthcare reform. Ann Health Law 1993;2:215–24.
15. Crossing the Quality Chasm: A New Health System for the 21st Century. Institute of Medicine. 2001. Available at: https://www.nationalacademies.org/hmd/Reports/2001/Crossing-the-Quality-Chasm-A-New-Health-System-for-the-21st-Century.aspx. Accessed February 2, 2017.
16. To Err is Human: Building a safer health system. Institute of Medicine. 1999. Available at: https://www.nationalacademies.org/hmd/Reports/1999/To-Err-is-Human-Building-A-Safer-Health-System.aspx. Accessed February 2, 2017.
17. Centers for Medicare and Medicaid Services. Hospital Outpatient Prospective Payment System. 2016. Available at: https://www.cms.gov/Outreach-and-Education/Medicare-Learning-Network-MLN/MLNProducts/downloads/Hospital Outpaysysfctsht.pdf. Accessed January 27, 2017.
18. Lindenauer PK, Remus D, Roman S, et al. Public reporting and pay for performance in hospital quality improvement. N Engl J Med 2007;256:486–96.
19. Stange KC, Nutting PA, Miller WL, et al. Defining and measuring the patient-centered medical home. J Gen Intern Med 2010;25:601–12.
20. Kash BS, Zhang Y, Cline KM, et al. The perioperative surgical home (PSH): a comprehensive review of US and non-US studies shows predominantly positive quality and cost outcomes. Milbank Q 2014;92(4):796–821.
21. Centers for Medicare & Medicaid Services. Bundled Payment Care Initiatives (BPCI). 2017. Available at: https://innovation.cms.gov/initiatives/bundled-payments/. Accessed January 18, 2017.

22. Health Care Center Incentives Improvement Institute. PROMETHEUS Payment. Available at: www.hci3.org/programs-efforts/prometheus-payment. Accessed on February 2, 2017.

23. Overland D. "BSBSNC bundles payments for better coordination, quality, costs." FierceHealthcare. 2013. Available at: www.fiercehealthcare.com/payer/bcbsnc-bundles-payments-for-better-coordination-quality-costs. Accessed February 2, 2017.

24. Centers for Medicare and Medicaid Services. Accountable Care Organizations. 2015. Available at: www.cms.gov/Medicare/Medicare-Fee-for-Service-Payment/ACO/index.html. Accessed January 19, 2017.

25. Centers for Medicare and Medicaid Services. Medicare shared savings program: accountable care organizations. Final Rule. Fed Regist 2011;76(212):67802–990.

26. Pham HH, Cohen M, Conway PH. The Pioneer accountable care organization model: improving quality and lowering costs. JAMA 2014;312(16):1635–6.

27. Centers for Medicare and Medicaid Services. Next Generation ACO Model. 2017. Available at: https://innovation.cms.gov/initiatives/Next-Generation-ACO-Model/. Accessed on January 18, 2017.

28. The Medicare Access and CHIP Reauthorization Act of 2015. HR 2. Available at: https://www.congress.gov/bill/114th-congress/house-bill/2. Accessed January 21, 2017.

29. Centers for Medicare and Medicaid Services. Comprehensive Care for Joint Replacement model. Available at: http://innovation.cms.gov/initiatives/ccjr/. Accessed January 21, 2017.

30. Rajkumar R, Conway PH, Tavvener M. CMS: engaging multiple payers in payment reform. JAMA 2014;311(19):1967–8.

31. Burwell SM. Setting value-based payment goals: HHS efforts to improve U.S. health care. N Engl J Med 2015;372(10):897–9.

Value-Based Care and Strategic Priorities

Wendy L. Gross, MD, MHCM[a,*], Lebron Cooper, MD[b], Steven Boggs, MD, MBA[b], Barbara Gold, MD, MS[c]

KEYWORDS

- Anesthesia • Market forces • Value-based care • Strategic priorities
- Strategic position • Financial silo(s) • Cost • Outcomes

KEY POINTS

- The anesthesia market continues to undergo disruption. Financial margins are shrinking, and buyers are demanding that anesthesia services are provided in an efficient, low-cost manner.
- Drucker and Porter's analysis of buyers, suppliers, quality, barriers to entry, substitution, and strategic priorities allows anesthesia groups to analyze their position in the market.
- To be operationally effective, anesthesiologists must articulate their value to other medical professionals and to hospitals seeking to only lower cost without considering other factors.
- Anesthesiologists can survive and thrive in a value-based health care environment if they are capable of providing services differently and able to deliver cost-effective care.

Fundamental tenets of finance, management, and strategic planning have become an integral part of infrastructure management and health care delivery. Efficient delivery of value-based care requires well-integrated operational systems. Alignment of goals and effort is difficult; the waters are choppy, and the weather is unpredictable. Politics and financial pressures are mounting as the population ages, technology expands, and financial coffers diminish. Competitive strategy remains siloed, but collaboration is increasingly necessary. Joint venture medicine and joint venture finance are likely to constitute the required platform for interdisciplinary practice.

Disclosure Statement: No disclosures for any authors.
[a] Division of Cardiac Anesthesia, Department of Anesthesiology, Perioperative and Pain Medicine, Brigham and Women's Hospital, 75 Francis Street, Boston, MA 02115, USA; [b] Department of Anesthesiology, University of Tennessee College of Medicine UTHSC/Regional One Health Chandler Building, Suite 600, 877 Jefferson Avenue, Memphis, TN 38103, USA; [c] Anesthesiology, Anesthesiology Administration, University of Minnesota Health, MMC 294 Mayo, 8294A (Campus Delivery Code), 420 Delaware Street Southeast, Minneapolis, MN 55455, USA
* Corresponding author.
E-mail address: WGROSS@partners.org

Anesthesiology Clin 35 (2017) 725–731
http://dx.doi.org/10.1016/j.anclin.2017.08.008
anesthesiology.theclinics.com

Businesses cannot succeed unless their goods and services reflect market needs, values, and behaviors. Success requires that there is adaptation to change, appropriate focusing of core competencies, and modification of perspective to include recognition and inclusion of disruptive technologies and paradigm shifts. Anesthesiology faces these challenges in the context of a churning health care marketplace.

THEORY OF THE BUSINESS

Establishing a mission based on accurate assessment of market forces and a clear honing of core competencies is required to execute the mission in an ongoing, dynamic process. The economic landscape is littered with failed businesses incapable of adaptation. The health care marketplace is subject to tectonic shifts. Successful compensation demands attention from medical practitioners, administrators, and financiers.

The core competencies of anesthesiologists include the performance of medical risk assessment, the development and execution of anesthetic plans based on the risks and goals of the procedure, and the implementation of pre-and postprocedure care regimens. In the operating room, anesthesiologists are necessary in order for patients to safely undergo surgical procedures; their periprocedural activities enhance efficiency and effectiveness. For these reasons, anesthesia care teams are highly valued in this environment. Core competencies effectively translate to environments outside the operating room. However, the procedures, degree of physiologic intrusion, and mindset of the providers with whom anesthesiologists work may be different from those in the operating room. The uniqueness and innovative character of the procedures may generate challenges that have not been encountered, and the operational platforms may be outside of managerial perimeters. It has become e clear over the past 5 years as the revenue streams generated by nonsurgical procedures rise,[1] that the need for patient risk assessment and efficiency has increased. Can anesthesiologists meet this need by lowering the threshold for discussion and negotiation between anesthesiologists and proceduralists, or will anesthesiologists force proceduralists to forge ahead without them and rely on the availability of code teams in the event of unanticipated problems?

Noninvasive procedures often invoke equal or higher- risk potentials than similarly focused surgeries. Lack of an incision does not automatically mitigate potential disaster, especially when the patient has been deemed too sick for surgery. Demand for anesthesiologists is often last minute; case rosters are often long and disorganized. Because investment in new technology is expensive, return on investment requires that interventionalists accomplish rapid turnover and high throughput. Target patient populations are unpredictable and include many with significant comorbidities. Preprocedural evaluation is inconsistent, making planning difficult.

If schedules were managed by anesthesiologists, relatively straightforward patients undergoing uncomplicated procedures could be properly delegated to trained sedation nurses. Patients with extensive comorbidities or complex procedures could be consistently assigned to anesthesia care teams. Of course, the most favorable condition would be for the highest level of evaluation to be available to all patients, but current operational platforms do not always allow this.

Anesthesiologists who can integrate their special competences in perioperative assessment with a thorough understanding of the procedures and the technologies being applied should attend to cases within their areas of expertise, just as they do in the operating room. Separating nonoperating room procedures into a bucket of cases attended by any and all anesthesia providers is inconsistent with an anesthesiologist's values and medical platforms. Accomplishing the mission and securing value outside of the operating room requires that anesthesiologists communicate with interventionists and learn the intricacies of new, noninvasive approaches to medical problems. For patients undergoing multiple procedures during 1 hospitalization, pre- and postprocedure care recommendations could be formulated by anesthesiologists in order to minimize length of stay and optimize outcomes, providing maximal value to patients and increasing financial sustainability for the institution. This is 1 example of how the anesthesiology theory of the business needs constant re-evaluation and reshaping in order to stay current with the health care marketplace.

Market Forces and Analysis

Just as strategic planning is required in the business world, it has become essential in medicine as well. Drucker and Porter[1,2] identified market forces critical to building effective competitive strategy. These are generated by buyers, suppliers, barriers to entry, the threat of substitutes, and potential rivalries.

Understanding and assessing these forces provide a useful framework for addressing a plan for development of anesthesia services in the nonoperating room environment and provides a useful framework for further analysis.

Buyers

The buyers of NORA services include hospital, proceduralists, and patients needing or seeking anesthesia services outside of the operating room. The power of a buying group is determined by its ability to demand high-quality or increased quantities of service at a lower price. Usually powerful buying groups are those with a large volume of business and needing standardized services that are easily acquired.

As disruptive innovation grows,[3] anesthesiologists must respond. As the numbers of nonoperating room cases increase, and buyers become more powerful within the hospital structure. Clearly, with respect to anesthesia services, quality is critical, and the product is not easily standardized, although this is often not apparent to proceduralists. In addition, although buyers feel that they are able to backward integrate (ie, perform the service themselves, via nurse-administered sedation, relying on code teams to perform a bailout if there is a problem), this will diminish as procedures become more technically demanding, and patient acuity rises. The threats of backward integration and of potentially high and increasing volume are obvious to the knowledgeable observer and have been documented in recent analyses.[4]

Suppliers

Suppliers within an industry are persons or organizations providing the resources needed to accomplish the mission at hand. If only a few suppliers provide a highly specialized resource, and the cost of switching suppliers is considerable, then suppliers occupy a dominant position. Clearly, the supply of specialized personnel to match the medical acuity of the situation is critical throughout the nonoperating room environment. Again, this is not always recognized by consumers of anesthesia services. The challenge is to reach agreement about the needs of the patient and to make proceduralists aware of the required level of involvement before disaster threatens. Financial and time constraints may have an inappropriate impact on such discussions. In the short term, a shortage of anesthesia personnel for staffing NORA procedures lowers the cost of switching to nonanesthesia personnel. This enhances fragmentation, which is not likely to be in anyone's best interest: anesthesiologists, proceduralists, or patients.[5]

Quality
Quality of service is hard to quantify unless there is a catastrophic bad outcome. Smaller problems are rarely documented, although electronic health records (EHRs) make it possible to find the data. Costs are difficult to tabulate. These include longer stays in recovery areas, unanticipated hospital admissions, and nonreimbursement of never events as defined by the Centers for Medicare and Medicaid Services (CMS). Electronic databases and ongoing required quality assessments by third-party payers are likely to improve the situation if the necessary information is recorded and available.

Barriers to entry
Barriers to entry into the nonoperating room market for anesthesiologists include the constant push for the use of propofol by individuals less skilled in airway management than anesthesiologists and the blurred continuum of care between moderate sedation, deep sedation, and general anesthesia. Increasing technical demands of non-operating room cases and higher acuity of nonoperating room patients oppose improvements in drug and monitoring. The expense of securing anesthesia providers imposes an additional barrier, but the opportunity for anesthesia personnel to contribute to the efficient care of these patients can also increase margin. This will increase the value of the anesthesia services to the hospital but not necessarily to the individual nonoperating room unit. The challenge is to identify new roles for anesthesiologists and to build a value-based financial platform that improves outcome, as discussed by Lee and Porter.[5] As some barriers are lowered, others arise. New skills will develop, and core competencies will expand in novel ways. The anesthesiologist's roles as integrators of services and purveyors of valued care have room to grow, and anesthesiologists will be asked to draw upon their medical backgrounds more frequently as proceduralists become more specialized and technologically oriented.

Substitution
An important market force that anesthesiologists must consider in nonoperating room areas is the use of a sedation nurse supervised by a proceduralist instead of an anesthesiologist, as well as the local-only option, in which no sedation is used. Although the anesthesia community may object to such alternatives, if there is no anesthesia care team available, and the proceduralist is willing to substitute another approach, then this becomes a viable alternative. Less optimal outcomes may not be immediately obvious, especially if the costs accrue elsewhere. This is the obvious danger; perceived substitutes may not be true substitutes. In this context, marketing, effective mutual communication, and transfer pricing become important issues.

Rivalry
The fifth market force that all businesses must contend with is internal rivalry. For example, a hospital may decide to backstop anesthesiologists in order to meet the needs of nonoperating room procedures, and support potential hospital margin. This limits the margin of anesthesia departments and relegates anesthesia departments to the land of cost centers. In some ways, proceduralists themselves are rivals, since they seek to develop budget-neutral approaches to interventions. However, the practice of assuming no need for anesthesia services may deliver suboptimal outcomes to patients and incur increased costs to hospitals. This sets the stage for rivalry and competition between anesthesia groups and interventionalists. Poor quality care will eventually result in lowered reimbursement, which benefits no one. The development of an informed competitive strategy will be stimulated by analysis of market

forces, consideration of anesthesia's theory of business, and consideration of business theory adaptation in the context of value-based care and new financial constructs within the health care marketplace.

STRATEGIC PRIORITIES

Hospitals and anesthesiologists understand the compelling need to extend modified operating room infrastructure to nonoperating room areas. This may require a new model of service delivery that includes new joint venture financial platforms. Not only are new procedural markets emerging,[3] but the financial rules are in flux.[5] Anesthesiologists are in danger of permitting their core competencies to fall out of step with market demands.

Disruptive technologies and noninvasive approaches to what were once purely surgical problems threaten to change the standards of care and challenge the rules of engagement.

The anesthesiologist's potential role in nonoperating room areas could revolutionize safety and everyone's scope of practice. The value of this is potentially enormous if it improves outcome and reduces cost. Consistent and continued assessments of value-based care, reorganization of nonoperating room areas into procedurally-based units, and parallel financial reorganization are critical to success. If anesthesiologists ignore these trends and the simultaneous emerging market demands, they abdicate their responsibility to patients and to medicine. Anesthesiologists need to define their goals in terms of the productivity and sustainability of anesthesiology as a medical subspecialty.

OPERATIONAL EFFECTIVENESS

Operational effectiveness is 1 component of competitive strategy and determines the profitability of all medical services. Innovation and adaptation to market conditions are critical. Anesthesiologists must successfully confront: medical proceduralists who believe they do not need an anesthesiologist and hospital administrators who do not recognize the value of anesthesia services. Innovation means providing flexible, adaptive services and techniques that can yield recognizably better outcomes. Better outcomes are defined by quality data and other forms of evidence; therefore, EHRs have become an essential element of operations. Operational effectiveness is achieved by well-planned active asset management using adequate information systems and high-quality database maintenance and analysis. It also requires awareness of changing practice landscapes on the part of leadership so that the perimeters of practice can advance. Performance frontiers move forward only if ongoing resource management is optimal and operationally effective.

VALUE, COST, AND OUTCOMES

Value-based health care is defined by improved outcome at reduced cost. Anesthesiologists will have the edge only if services are provided differently, more cost-effectively, and with better results than the existing, or potential competition can provide them.

Is maintaining the edge possible, given changing reimbursement strategies, bundling tactics, and potential CMS reforms? Accurate cost accounting across departmental cost centers is necessary to understand the financial implications and necessary reforms.

The expense incurred by delaying a case, stopping a procedure due to inadequate sedation, unanticipated hospitalization, and redoing the procedure is often hidden by financial silos. The cost of pulling an anesthesiologist from another location is high, but the cost of a bad outcome is far higher.

The contexts in which anesthesiologists practice, and the medical and surgical departments they serve, benefit from their services. However, reimbursement to anesthesiologists in nonoperating room arenas is often inadequate, because inefficiency is widespread. The benefits of improved quality of care accrue to other departments and to the hospital.

STRATEGIC POSITION

Strategic positioning should reflect the needs of customers, potential customers, and market shifts.[6] This essentially means reconciling the theory of the business with revision of core competencies and the results of environmental scanning and context analysis. Customers include patients, medical proceduralists, and third-party payers. When industries get into trouble it is usually because products and services are out of sync with market demands. Hence, anesthesiologists must revise their core competencies to ensure that noncustomers become customers and that value is clear. If anesthesiologists can demonstrate that they provide a safer, more comfortable, and more time-efficient environment for interventional medicine procedures, and they have the data to prove that they do, then the value of an anesthesiologist in attendance becomes unmistakable. Not only does it become clear to proceduralists and patients, it also becomes clear to payors, regulatory bodies, and government agencies.

TEAMWORK AND FINANCIAL SILOS

As bundling becomes standard, and integration becomes a factor of value-based care, anesthesiologists will come to rely on the strength of medical, interpersonal, and financial relationships forged between themselves and medical specialists. These relationships can grow and develop only as medical specialists witness and comprehend the value of anesthesiologists to their practices. Team building improves outcomes but requires communication, common language, and common goals. Hence the argument for creating integrated practice groups that have consistent goals and common financial and medical practice platforms.

KEY ELEMENTS OF SUSTAINABLE STRATEGY

The goal of any strategy is to maintain a dynamic and profitable market presence in the context of current demands and market projections. In health care, this means providing highly valued care that delivers optimized outcomes. Anesthesiologists have several parallel sets of priorities:

- Creating and maintaining a stable but flexible customer base
- Facilitating optimal outcomes
- Achieving financial sustainability

Appropriate resource allocation promotes innovation. Enhanced core competencies resulting from expanded nonoperating room experience can provide enriched services. Team building solidifies the rationale for collaboration and helps to create a mutually acceptable platform for joint venture finance. Eradication of fragmented care can improve quality, reduce cost, and enhance value. Anesthesiologists' expertise will justify reliable and sustained reimbursement if they have the data to demonstrate the benefit of that presence. Anesthesiologists' participation in nonoperating room venues can stimulate and advance medicine just as their position in the operating room advanced the practice of surgery. As technology continues to proliferate and diversify, anesthesiologists have seen the proliferation of noninvasive techniques in nonoperating room arenas. Only by remaining innovative and building collaborative bridges can anesthesiology maintain its position as a respected medical subspecialty.

Anesthesiology is challenged by dynamic market forces. There is an urgent need for anesthesiologists to engage a broad business-like perspective, to reassess their market, mission, and core competencies. If anesthesiologists ignore this responsibility, their very status as a medical subspecialty may be threatened. If anesthesiologists accept it, they will help to define the front lines of the medical horizon.

REFERENCES

1. Peter D. Theory of the business. Harvard Business Review 1994.
2. Porter M. What is strategy? Harvard Business Review 1996.
3. Bower J, Christenson C. Disruptive technologies: catching the wave. Harvard Business Review 1995.
4. Nagrebetsky A, Gabriel RA, Dutton RP, et al. Growth of nonoperating room anesthesia care in the United States: a contemporary trends analysis. Anesth Analg 2017;124(4):1261–7.
5. Lee T, Porter M. The strategy that will fix healthcare. Harvard Business Review 2013.
6. Porter M. How competitive forces shape strategy. Harvard Business Review 1979.

Printed and bound by CPI Group (UK) Ltd, Croydon, CR0 4YY

08/05/2025

01864701-0003